Nada Yoga

of related interest

Yoga Teaching Handbook
A Practical Guide for Yoga Teachers and Trainees
Edited by Sian O'Neill
ISBN 978 1 84819 355 0
eISBN 978 0 85701 313 2
Yoga Teaching Guides

Holding Space
The Creative Performance and Voice Workbook for Yoga Teachers
Sarah Scharf, MFA
Foreword by Judith Hanson Lasater, Ph.D., P.T.
ISBN 978 1 84819 405 2
eISBN 978 0 85701 361 3

Water Yoga
A Teacher's Guide to Improving Movement, Health and Wellbeing
Christa Fairbrother
Foreword by Ruth Sova
ISBN 978 1 83997 285 0
eISBN 978 1 83997 286 7

Restorative Yoga
Power, Presence and Practice for Teachers and Trainees
Anna Ashby
Foreword by Richard Rosen
ISBN 978 1 78775 739 4
eISBN 978 1 78775 740 0

Yoga Therapy as a Whole-Person Approach to Health
Lee Majewski and Ananda Balayogi Bhavanani
Foreword by Stephen Parker
ISBN 978 1 78775 092 0
eISBN 978 1 78775 093 7

NADA YOGA

The Vibratory Essence of the Yoga of Sound

Dr. Sangeeta Laura Biagi
Dr. Ananda Balayogi Bhavanani

Foreword by Rajiv Mehrotra

Illustrations by Yogacharini Padma and Sri M Sridharan

SINGING DRAGON
LONDON AND PHILADELPHIA

First published in Great Britain in 2024 by Singing Dragon,
an imprint of Jessica Kingsley Publishers
Part of John Murray Press

1

A CIP catalogue record for this title is available from the
British Library and the Library of Congress

ISBN 978 1 83997 450 2
eISBN 978 1 83997 451 9

Printed and bound in Great Britain by TJ Books Limited

Jessica Kingsley Publishers' policy is to use papers that are natural, renewable and recyclable
products and made from wood grown in sustainable forests. The logging and manufacturing
processes are expected to conform to the environmental regulations of the country of origin.

Singing Dragon
Carmelite House
50 Victoria Embankment
London EC4Y 0DZ

www.singingdragon.com

John Murray Press
Part of Hodder & Stoughton Limited
An Hachette UK Company

FSC www.fsc.org
MIX
Paper from
responsible sources
FSC® C013056

Contents

Illustration List

Yogacharini Padma:

- Nada, Bindu, Kala
- Vibhaga Pranayama Inhalation
- Vibhaga Pranayama Exhalation
- Pranava Pranayama Inhalation/Mahat Yoga Pranayama Inhalation
- Pranava Pranayama Exhalation/Mahat Yoga Pranayama Exhalation
- Evolution of Tattwas
- Pinda Chakras, Bija, and Tattwas

Sri M Sridharan (Brushline Graphtech):

- Vibhaga Pranayama Hasta Mudras
- Nadis and Chakras
- Pinda Chakras/Anda Chakras
- The Petals of Sahasrara
- Adhi-Vyadhi

FOREWORD

I am blessed to introduce *Nada Yoga: The Vibratory Essence of the Yoga of Sound*. Co-authored by Yogacharya Dr. Ananda Balayogi Bhavanani and Yogacharini Dr. Sangeeta Laura Biagi, the book is more than just a collection of how-to drills. It offers a wealth of theoretical and contextual information, a scholarly contribution to the rich repertoire of writings that enrich the contemporary discourse and understanding of Yoga.

The authors epitomize in their lives and work the aspiration to revive the rich tradition of Yoga in all of its intricacies, subtleties, and richness. They have reached far beyond the narrow contemporary perspective of Yoga as mere asana to nurture its diverse aspects. They achieve this by expanding their boundaries and evolving numerous practice protocols without jeopardizing their authenticity, impacting thousands to live healthy and fulfilling lives.

Ananda was born in an ashram to Yogamaharishi Swami Gitananda Giri, the inheritor of the ancient lineage of the Gurus of the Kambaliswamy Madam tradition, and his wife, Yogacharini Meenakshi Devi. He brings to bear the rich Parampara of his parents' Gurukul and a lineage that goes back for hundreds of years. His parents were among my first Gurus.

Dr. Sangeeta Laura Biagi adopted the same lineage and is an accomplished researcher, artist, and International Director of Gitananda Nada Yoga. Her work explores the human voice in interpersonal, intrapersonal, and transpersonal relationships.

Dr. Bhavanani and Dr. Biagi draw on teachings from the Yogamaharishi Swami Gitananda Giri tradition. His teachings have profoundly impacted many lives, and I am pleased to see his wisdom shared through this book. The authors have done an excellent job of explaining complex concepts in a way that is accessible to all readers. Drawing upon their extensive knowledge of Indian philosophy, Yoga, and music, they offer a wealth of insights and practical exercises designed to help readers deepen their understanding of Nada Yoga's transformative potential.

The ancient Indian practice of Nada Yoga, also known as the Yoga of Sound, has gained popularity as a powerful method of self-realization and spiritual development in recent years. At its core, it entails tuning in to the music playing inside one's head. These vibrations, produced by the movement of energy in our bodies, constitute the very essence of life. By working with external sounds that resonate with these vibrations within us, we can tune into them to promote physical and mental well-being.

The book points to its potential in the spiritual quest by exploring the concept of the Pranava Aum, considered the primordial sound that gave birth to the universe. Tracing its roots back to ancient Indian texts such as the *Upanishads* and the *Bhagavad Gita*, the authors delve into the significance of sonic vibrations in religions like Hinduism, Buddhism, and Sufism. The authors examine how chanting Aum can help individuals connect with their inner selves and the universe, how sound vibration cultivates awareness of both the divine and the self, and how Nada Yoga can help us connect with a more profound sense of spirituality.

One of its intriguing components is the idea of "anahata nada," or the unstruck sound. The internal music constantly plays, which the external din often obscures. As the authors describe, Nada Yoga helps us tune in to that quiet, steady voice within, bringing us closer to our authentic selves and fostering a sense of inner serenity.

Providing a range of exercises that readers can practice daily, the book offers guidance on using our voice, breath, and musical instruments to create and manipulate sound to nurture spiritual well-being. It has specific advice on incorporating vibrations into one's meditative practices, asana practice, as it discusses the body's chakras, or energy centers, and how sound vibrations can stimulate these.

The authors also explain the role of yoga music therapies in promoting salutogenesis, which is the process of maintaining and enhancing health. Through summaries of research studies, they demonstrate sound therapy's efficacy in treating various health conditions, including stress, anxiety, and depression.

Drawing upon their own experiences as Nada Yoga practitioners and instructors, Bhavanani and Biagi share stories and anecdotes illustrating the transformative power and the deep sense of peace and joy the practice offers. To invite readers to experience the healing power of sound, there is also a selection of Mantras and Bhajans from Ananda Ashram, founded by Swami Gitananda.

Nada Yoga: The Vibratory Essence of the Yoga of Sound is a comprehensive and insightful guide to the practice of Nada Yoga. The authors' deep knowledge and passion for the subject shine through in every chapter, and readers are sure to come away with a greater understanding of the power of sound vibrations and their potential for transformation and healing. Whether you are a seasoned practitioner of Nada Yoga or just starting on your journey, this book will surely be an invaluable resource.

Rajiv Mehrotra
Hon. Trustee and Secretary
The Foundation for Universal Responsibility of His Holiness the Dalai Lama

Acknowledgments

We are indeed blessed to be Sishyas (śiṣya) of the Great Rishiculture Guru Parampara (paramparā) and express our gratitude to our illustrious Gurus Yogamaharishi Dr. Swami Gitananda Giri Guru Maharaj and Param Pujya Ammaji Yogacharini Smt Meenakshi Devi Bhavanani who have blessed us with this life of Yoga. They are the light onto Yoga for us and are the causative energies enlightening anything we have of worth in this lifetime.

We offer this book as our loving gratitude and dedication to Parampujya Ammaji who is truly the Living Siddha of Pondicherry. Her life of Yoga is one of Divinity and blesses us all with wisdom, grace, beauty, and love.

We acknowledge the Gurus of this lineage and, in particular, Swami Purnananda Brighu, Swami Vivideshananda Brighu, Swami Kanakananda Brighu, and Srila Sri Shankara Giri Swamigal. May their blessings continue to shower us with grace, strength, and compassion.

We acknowledge with gratitude the loving teachings of the illustrious Natya and Sangeeta Gurus of the Rishiculture Parampara, namely the unparalleled Natya Guru Padmashri Adyar K Lakshmanan, Puduvai Kalaimamani Srirengam R Ranganathan, Puduvai Kalaimamani V Manikannan, Tiruvaroor Sri R Krishnamurthy, Thamizhmamani Pulavar I Pattabiramane, and Sangeeta Kalanidhi Padmabhushan TV Sankaranarayanan, who have been a major source of inspiration in our lives. They have been living legends of Nada Yoga; indeed, human incarnations of its complete wholesomeness.

We thank all our elders, families, friends, well-wishers, and colleagues who have been a major support in this initiative. Each and every one of these true human beings is an inspiration for us and they motivate us to do our best at all times through their constant feedback and encouragement. They are perfect examples of the qualities extolled by Maharishi Patanjali: being friendly towards those at ease with themselves and being cheerful towards the virtuous (maitrī-sukha mudita-puṇya).

We thank all the Gitananda Yoga Mentors around the world for sharing the teachings of this tradition far and wide and for supporting each other and our students.

We thank all of our students and, in particular, the students who enrolled in our online and residential Nada Yoga courses and provided feedback, inspiration, and new insights.

In particular, for transcribing a selection of online lessons by Dr. Ananda and Dr. Sangeeta, we thank Yogacharya Bharata Bill Francis Barry, Hwamin Fettes, Valananda Joyce, Antonio Manzionna, Michael McCann, Amanda Paulson, and Ovidiu Ciprian Ponoran.

A special note of gratitude for Yogacharya Bharata Bill Francis Barry for the meticulous work of proofreading the first draft of the manuscript and providing suggestions and changes that made the manuscript clearer and more precise. Our gratitude to Yogasadhaka Nilachal for proofing the Sanskrit quotations and transliterations, Antonio Manzionna for offering constructive feedback on the book's "strong points," Yoga Thilakam Dr. Meena Ramanathan for constructive feedback on the chapter on Yoga Chikitsa, and Judith Moloney for editing the bibliography. We would also like to thank Yogacharini Devasena Bhavanani, Dhivya Priya Bhavanani, Yogacharini Kalavathi Devi, Yogacharini Anandhi-Korina Kontaxaki, Mario Biagi, Giuliana Manganelli, Stefania Biagi, Matilde Rossi, Ilaria Biagi, Ilaria Fiorenzani, Chiara Iacomelli, and Abigail Hendricks for supporting us during various phases of this project. Last but not least, we thank our brilliant illustrators, Yogacharini Padma and Sri M Sridharan, for providing visuals that not only illustrate words but elucidate certain concepts even more than words could.

A Note on Sanskrit

Sanskrit (saṃskṛta) is a system of communication that was heard, Shruti (śruti), by the sages of ancient India before its phonemes were written down. It is considered to be the "language of the Gods," Devanagari (devanāgarī), and it is the language of Yoga (yoga). The lineage of Yogamaharishi Dr. Swami Gitananda Giri is committed to employing Sanskrit terms in teachings, research papers, and talks. For this book, the authors made the decision to include the Sanskrit terms employed in this tradition and to write them with a capitalized English transliteration followed, when first appearing in the text, by a transliteration with diacritical marks in parenthesis for correct pronunciation. Direct quotes of teachings from the *Vedas*, the *Upanishads* (upaniṣad), the *Bhagavad Gita* (bhagavadgītā), the *Yoga Sutra* (yoga sūtra), and the *Hatha Yoga Pradipika* (haṭha yoga pradīpikā), to name a few, appear in Devanagari script, followed by a transliteration with diacritical marks.

Sanskrit Pronunciation

Classical Sanskrit has at least 49 letters: 14 vowels, 33 consonants, and two special letters. Four additional letters are occasionally used. Supplements are required because the 26 letters of the Roman alphabet are insufficient to express all of Sanskrit's sounds. One Roman letter is used to represent one Sanskrit sound whenever possible. Otherwise, two Roman letters are combined to represent one Sanskrit sound (such as the vowels ai and au and the ten aspirated consonants), or a Roman letter with a diacritical mark. Six diacritics are used in Sanskrit romanization:

- a line above the letter (ā)

- a line below the letter (ḻ)
- a dot above the letter (ṅ)
- a dot below the letter (ḍ)
- a tilde or curl above the letter (ñ)
- an acute accent above the letter (ś).

The following points will enable you to learn the pronunciation of most transliterated Sanskrit terms and Mantras:

Vowels

The vowels are: *a, ā, i, ī, u, ū, ṛ, ṝ, ḷ, ḹ, e, ai, o, au*. Vowels are pronounced *a* [a], *i* [ee], *u* [oo], *ṛ* and *ḷ* [these two vowels are cerebral retroflex sounds made by curling the tongue towards the area between the alveolar ridge and the "soft" palate], *e* [è] like the sound of *e* in "helicopter," *ai* [aee], *o* [ow] as in the beginning of "ow-n," and *au* [a+oo].

The journey of the vowels in the oral cavity goes from the guttural resonance at the bottom of the throat, to the palatal resonance at the back of the throat/palate, to the cerebral resonance in the roof of the oral cavity.

A line over one of a pair of vowels distinguishes long from short. Vowels with a dash above them (ā, ī, ū, ṝ, ḹ) take about twice as long to pronounce as their short counterparts (*a, i, u, ṛ, ḷ*). Pronounce the vowels as follows:

- *ā* (long) is like the *a* in father, as in māyā (illusion)
- *i* (short) is like the *i* in pin, as in idam (this)
- *ī* (long) is like the *i* in pique, as in jīva (life)
- *u* (short) is like the *u* in put, as in guṇa (quality)
- *ū* (long) is like the *u* in rune, as in rūpa (form)
- *ṛ* (short) is often pronounced *ri*, as in the name Kṛṣṇa or Krishna
- *ṝ* (long) is like the re in fiber, as in pitṝṇām (of the fathers)
- *ḷ* (short) is like the *le* in able, as in the root kḷp.

The following four vowels are always long in Sanskrit:

- *e* is like the *ei* in rein, as in deva (god) (note: Sanskrit *e* is never short like the *e* in yet)
- *ai* is like the *ai* in aisle, as in vaiśya (merchant) (note: Sanskrit *ai* is never like the *ai* in pain)
- *o* is like the *o* in opal, as in loka (world) (note: Sanskrit *o* is never short like the *o* in pot)
- *au* is like the *ou* in out, as in Gautama Buddha (note: Sanskrit *au* is never like the *au* in autumn).

Consonants

(The sound of A is added to the sound of the consonants, as in *k* [ka].)

Sanskrit has 33 consonants, divided into eight groups, and two special letters, as shown below with the grammatical name for each group in Sanskrit order.

- Guttural consonants: *k*, *kh*, *g*, *gh*, *n*; *k* [ka as in "car"], *g* [ga as in "garage"], *ṅ* [this sound does not have an exact equivalent in English but you can imagine you are making the sound of N from your throat].
- Palatal consonants: *c*, *ch*, *j*, *jh*, *ñ*; *c* is pronounced similarly to the "ch" in choice; *j* [*ja* as in "Jack"]; *ñ* [this sound does not have an exact equivalent in English; make the sound of N by flattening the body of the tongue in the front area of your palate].
- Retroflex consonants: *ṭ*, *ṭh*, *ḍ*, *ḍh*, *ṇ*; these sounds have no exact equivalent in English; they are pronounced like the dentals *t, th, d, dh,* and *n,* except that for retroflex letters the tip of the tongue is bent back to touch the roof of the mouth—the area between the alveolar ridge and the "soft" palate—while for dentals the tongue touches the teeth.
- Dental consonants: *t*, *th*, *d*, *dh*, *n*.
- Labial consonants: *p*, *ph*, *b*, *bh*, *m*.
- The semivowels are *y* (palatal), *r* (retroflex), *l* (dental), *v* (labial).
- Sibilants are *ś* (palatal), *ṣ* (retroflex), *s* (dental); *ś* and *ṣ* produce sounds

similar to the English "sh" in shine and are often written as "sh" in English. The first, ś, is a palatal sound in which the back of the tongue touches the soft palate. The second, ṣ, is a cerebral sound produced by a "rounding" of the tongue closer to the floor of the oral cavity. Examples include śūdra (servant), puruṣa (person), śiṣṭa (residue).

- Aspirate: All consonants followed by an "*h*" are aspirated: *kh*, *gh*, *ch*, *jh*, *ṭh*, *ḍh*, *th*, *dh*, *ph*, *bh*. *Th* and *ṭh* are pronounced like the "t" in "target" and the "tr" in "trap," respectively, not like the "th" in "the." The *ph* is pronounced like the "p" in "partial," not like the "ph" in "pharaoh."

Pronounce the following consonants as in English:

- *b* as in buddha (awakened)
- *d* as in deva (god)
- *j* as in jīva (life)
- *k* as in karman (action)
- *l* as in loka (world)
- *m* as in manas (mind)
- *n* as in nivṛtti (involution)
- *p* as in pitṛ (father)
- *r* as in rūpa (form)
- *s* as in sat (reality)
- *t* as in tat (that).

Visarga

ḥ, the visarga, is an aspiration at the end of certain words ending in a vowel, either at the end of a word or before a consonant. This sound is subtle; for example: duḥkha (suffering) or namaḥ (homage).

Anuswara

Anuswara (anusvāra) is written *ṃ or ṁ*, a nasal-cerebral "m." A simple rule is to pronounce it as *m* at the end of a word or before *p, ph, b, bh*, or an other *m*, and otherwise as *n*. Anuswara stands for a nasal sound pronounced in one of three ways:

- at the end of a word, as *m*
- before semivowels *y, r, l, v*, sibilants *ś, ṣ, s*, and the aspirate *h*, as a nasalized vowel (as in French *bon*)
- before other consonants, as the nasal consonant of the same group; thus ahaṃkāra (egoism) may be written ahaṃkāra, and sannyāsin (renouncer) may be written saṃnyāsin.

Note: Anuswara has other linguistic rules and variations in sound but this detailed information is not necessary for the purpose of this book.

INTRODUCTION

The Parampara of Yogamaharishi
Dr. Swami Gitananda Giri Guru Maharaj

The Source

The Yoga Parampara of ICYER at Ananda Ashram Pondicherry, South India, is the Rishiculture Ashtanga Yoga (ṛṣi-culture aṣṭāṅga yoga) as synthesized by Yogamaharishi Dr. Swami Gitananda Giri (1907–1993). The rich Vedic Rishi concepts and practices, which contain the ones included in this book, were received by Yogamaharishi Dr. Swami Gitananda Giri from his Ashtanga Yoga Master Sri Swami (svāmī) Kanakananda Brighu, a Bengali saint, who initiated Swami Gitananda (then Ananda Bhavanani) at the age of ten years into this ancient Yoga teaching in Swamiji's[1] ancestral childhood home in Maharajganj, Bihar. Swami Gitananda maintained his relationship with his Guru, who lived in Swamiji's ancestral home, until Swami Kanakananda's Samadhi (samādhi) on October 26, 1967.

Swami Kanakananda was Professor in the Central Hindu College that later became the Banaras Hindu University in the early 1900s. Tragedy struck in his life when a disastrous fire destroyed the Varanasi housing colony in which he lived with his wife and infant son. Both his wife and son died in the fire. Driven nearly insane by the tragedy, Ram Gopal Majumdar (as he was then known) ran away into the Himalayas to wander as a Sadhu (sādhu), seeking peace of the soul. In the course of his Parivrajaka (pārivrājaka), "the life of a religious mendicant," he met Swami Vivideshananda Bhrigu, who

1 Swami/Swamiji is how Yogamaharishi Dr. Swami Gitananda Giri Guru Maharaj is addressed by his family members and his students.

initiated him into a particularly rich Yoga tradition, which contained Asanas (āsana, postures), Pranayamas (prāṇāyāma, breath and energy control), and Dharana (dhāraṇa, concentration) practices. Swami Vivideshananda had learned this esoteric knowledge from his Guru, Swami Purnananda Bhrigu, who was part of a long line of Yoga Gurus. Thus, the transformation from mathematics professor to saint occurred.

At the age of 16, Swami Gitananda moved to England to study medicine and then traveled to North and South America and settled in Canada. He was a pioneer of the movement in which the teachings of the East percolated to the West. In 1967 Swami Kanakananda left his body, and his last request to Swami Gitananda was that he return to India to take over his work, which he did in December of that year. He established Ananda Ashram in central Pondicherry and visited all the holy places in and around Pondicherry at that time to offer his Pranams (praṇam, devoted salutations) to the Great Souls who had hallowed this land.

At that time, he had visited a small Madam, a sacred site set in a jungle-like environment in Thattanchavady on the northwestern side of Pondicherry, far past the luscious rice lands and village tanks that then flourished there. He met the old Sadhu in charge, Srila Sri Shankara Giri Swamigal, who told him of the great power of the shrine of Sri Swamy, whose Samadhi was at the center of the Madam. Sri Kambaliswamigal was a Digambari Sannyasin who took Jala (jāla) Samadhi in the Amavasi of Marghazhi in 1863. Sri Kambaliswamigal was a great Siddha, and many miracles are attributed to him. He was praised in many old beautiful Tamil hymns as The King of Ashtanga Yoga over the whole Earth. He was also hailed as a Kalpa Vriksha (vṛkṣa) who would grant all boons of his devotees. Other hymns declared he was worthy of worship by the whole world. At that time, the Madam consisted of one small, tiled house, and the Samadhi of Sri Kambaliswamigal. Few dared to venture there, as it was infested with cobras and scorpions and the land behind it was used as a cemetery, but Swami Gitananda was attracted to the Samadhi and to the Sadhu, whom he visited often. Swamiji established Ananda Ashram in October 1969 in Lawspet, which was only a half-kilometer walk from Sri Kambaliswamy Madam. He then began to frequently visit and participate in all spiritual activities there.

During the Annual Guru Puja (pūjā, ritual practices) in December 1973, Srila Shri Shankara Giri, then 73 years of age, fell ill and requested Swami Gitananda to perform the Pujas. On January 21, 1975, Srila Shri Shankara

Giri nominated Swami Gitananda as his legal heir and successor to the position of Hereditary Trustee and Madathipathi of Sri Kambaliswamy Madam as per the Madam tradition. Then began the great restoration and rebuilding of Sri Kambaliswamy Madam by Swami Gitananda. The Madam became famous throughout India and the world as an ideal Guru Kula ("womb" and home of the Guru) and a Shanti (śānti) Niketan, "abode of peace," in South India. Classes in Ashtanga Yoga, Bharatanatyam (bharatanāṭyam), and Carnatic vocal music started in 1975 and attracted thousands of local and international students.

Srila Sri Shankara Giri Swamigal was a Siddha, who lived the life of a traditional Sannyasi (saṃnyāsin). Born in a village near Trichy, into a family of goldsmiths, he renounced the world at the age of 51 and spent nearly a decade wandering in the Himalayas. He came to Kambaliswamy Madam in the early 1960s and became the chief disciple of Subramaniya Giri Swamigal, then head of the Madam. He became well known as an adept in Siddha medicine and many Siddha medicinal herbs were grown in the Madam. He was named as successor to Subramaniya Giri Swamigal.

Sri Shankara Giri wore his hair coiled on top of his head and, when he opened the coil, his hair was more than five meters in length. He was born on December 25, 1900, and lived a very austere, simple life, walking wherever he went, sometimes as much as 50 kilometers a day. He was a staunch upholder of Dharma (dharma), and his favorite saying was: "Dharma protects those who protect Dharma." He had a great influence on Ananda Balayogi, son of Sri Swami Gitananda, and confirmed young Ananda as the successor and head of Sri Kambaliswamy Madam in January 1994. Srila Sri Shankara Giri Swamigal was the Chief Guest for many Ananda Ashram programs even though he was then in his nineties; he relished each and every program and gave his perceptive remarks and appreciation for all of them. Shankara Giri Swamigal attained Mukti on June 11, 1995, at the age of 95. His Samadhi is in the western side of Sri Kambaliswamy Madam, and daily Pujas are performed there.

Thus, the Rishiculture Ashtanga Yoga teachings of Sri Kanakananda Swamigal and the South Indian Saiva Siddhanta (śaiva siddhānta) tradition of Akanda Paripurna Srila Sri Jnanananda Desigar Kambaliswamigal came together in Yogamaharishi Dr. Swami Gitananda Giri Guru Maharaj, and the spirits of these great Gurus are the guiding force behind all of the activities of the present Ananda Ashram.

Yogacharya Dr. Ananda Balayogi Bhavanani (Giri) is the current lineage holder of the Rishiculture Gitananda Yoga tradition and current Madathipathi of the Sri Kambaliswamy Madam. He continues the illustrious tradition under the watchful guidance of his mother, Puduvai Kalaimamani Puduvai Shakti, Yogacharini Meenakshi Devi Bhavanani, Pujya Ammaji, one of the great Yoginis of Modern Times. Dr. Ananda lives and shares his Dharma with his wife (dharmapatnī), Yogacharini Devasena Bhavanani, an accomplished Natyacharini and Sangeeta Vidhushi, supported ably by their daughter, Dhivya Priya Bhavanani, and son, Anandraj Bhavanani.

Core Concepts of Rishiculture Ashtanga (Gitananda) Yoga

Before we delve deeper into the teachings of Nada Yoga (nāda yoga), we would like to share some core concepts of Rishiculture Ashtanga Yoga to start our journey:

Yoga is a Way of Life

Yoga is a Sanskrit term whose etymology comes from the Sanskrit Yuj (yuj), "to unite, to blend, to make whole." The root of the word has three meanings, according to the grammar of Maharshi Pāṇini: 1. Rudhādiganiya, which means unification or union; 2. Churādiganiya, which means to control the mind; and 3. Diwādiganiya, which means samādhi (ultimate liberation from the bondage of ignorance).

On the basis of its origin from the root Yuj, the word Yoga means "union, restraint of mind, and samādhi," and therefore, Yoga is not something we "do," but rather, Yoga is a way of life. Understanding this difference is of great importance because Yoga is both the goal of the practices (union with all that is, i.e., becoming one with pure consciousness) and the process that attains the goal. Yoga as a process involves a conscious transformation from a state of "doing" to a state of "being." This requires immense introspection, consciousness, awareness, dedication, and determination. Many will exclaim that this is easy to say and tough to do but Swami Gitananda "walked his talk" and showed us how to do it by his magnificent example.

In the principles and practices of Nada Yoga, a conscious state of Yoga is attained through deep listening to inner and outer sounds, from the metaphysical cosmic vibration, to the physical and physiological attunement to one's heartbeat. Yoga is an uninterrupted state of awareness that we are One with the Source of all that is, that Ultimate undivided intelligence that sustains the laws of the Universe. Considering that everything in our cosmos is moving and vibrating, from the atoms that sustain our body to the furthest galaxies, Nada Yoga is a process of merging with the resonance of that Divine Source.

Breath is Life

There is no life without breath! Swamiji was truly a grand master of this intricate and detailed science of subtle energy. In this tradition, great emphasis is placed on learning how to breathe properly, and the students start with the sectional breathing of Vibhaga Pranayama (vibhāga prāṇāyāma) and then build up step by step to the knowledge and practice of more than 120 intricate Pranayamas. All of this is done so that Prana (prāṇa), the vital cosmic catalyst, may naturally fill each and every one of our trillions of cells with life and light.

This teaching is even more important for those who are naturally drawn to the practices of Nada Yoga because the sound of our breath is a powerful Mantra that we repeat, consciously or unconsciously, over 21,600 times per day. The sound of the movement of energy of our inhalation and exhalation is the Ajapa Japa Mantra (ajapā japa mantra) "Soham" (sohaṃ). The definition of the word Mantra (mantra) in Sanskrit is "mananāt trāyatē iti mantrah": "sustained repetition (mananāt) of that which protects (trāyatē) from all miseries arising from bondage or cycles from birth and death is called mantra" (Parthasarathi, 2020, p.84). In Nada Yoga practices, we connect with our breath as a vehicle for our voice to teach, chant, recite, invoke, sing, and, most importantly, listen.

No Option Yoga

Swamiji termed Maharishi Patanjali's (maharṣi patañjali) Ashtanga Yoga (aṣṭāṅga yoga) the "No Option Yoga" and placed great importance on the study and understanding of the Yamas (yama, moral constraints) and Niyamas (niyama, ethical precepts), which are the firm foundation upon which the real Yoga life can be built. "You wouldn't build a colossal building without a foundation but you want to do it with Yoga?" he would ask numerous easy-going aspirants who wanted some "quick fix" Yoga.

Step-by-Step Approach

Every aspect of Swamiji's teachings follows a step-by-step, structured approach that is easy to follow, detailed, and methodical. Emphasis is placed on learning and relearning the preceding steps until the teachings are well digested, before proceeding any further on the path. "No shortcuts please" was his constant refrain, for it is always better to be slow and steady than fast and sorry. Great emphasis is placed on growing into the practice rather than forcing oneself into it, thus enabling growth to occur at all levels.

Love for Indian Culture

One of the major issues facing Yoga in the West is the fact that Yoga has been cleaved away from Indian culture (sanātana dharma, the eternal law). Without an understanding of Indian culture, it may be difficult to find answers for many questions confronting the sincere seeker. Swamiji tried to inculcate in his students a deep love and understanding of the ancient living culture from which Yoga has sprung.

Bountiful Practices

Scores and scores of practices and techniques are part of this tradition that has numerous Hatha (haṭha), Laya (laya), and Jnana (jñāna) Yoga practices for the sincere aspirant. Polarity practices and the Mantra Laya (mantra laya) deserve special mention, as do the Laya Yoga Kriyas (laya yoga kriyā). The intricate and in-depth understanding of Nadis (nāḍī) and Bindus (bindu) of the twelve Chakras (cakra) and Mantra Yoga shared in this book is gleaned from the Dakshina Marga Tantra (dakṣiṇa mārga tantra) tradition of Yogamaharishi Swami Kanakananda Brighu and are not found elsewhere. Each of these practices and concepts has multiple levels for the sincere seeker, and those who have gone deep into them understand that they are not mere playthings but are indeed very powerful and life transforming.

Tantra, Mantra, and Yantra: "In Tune" with Nature

In this Parampara there are three important sciences, namely Tantra (tantra), Mantra, and Yantra (yantra). Tantra is a Yoga philosophy and practical understanding of reality in which our inner and outer worlds coincide and influence each other. Tantra provides a practical map of the matrix of existence and focuses on the movement of subtle energies in our various bodies (physical, physiological, energetic, emotional, mental, and spiritual), in our environment, and in the multiverse in which we live.

Mantra is the study and practice of the vibration of such energies, from the mental vibrations of thought to the material utterances of our vocal apparatus. Mantras are poetic invocations in Vedic and ancient Sanskrit that have been perceived by the saintly Rishis (ṛṣi) of India thanks to the refinement of their clairaudience. The Rishis organized and passed down the Mantras in the complex oral system of the four *Vedas* (veda), which only later were written down. Mantras help us relax and focus the mind, quiet down destructive thinking, and invoke and evoke the power of love as it manifests through the elements and their essential forces, their "seed sounds," the Bija Mantras (bīja mantra).

Yantra is the mystical science of number, name, and form and is a method by which one can learn to live "in tune" with the cycles of the Universe rather than be "off tune" with those very cycles. According to the Yantra concepts taught by Swamiji, each number has a special quality to it and is not merely a measure of quantity as is usually presumed. Every aspect of life goes through a "phase of Nine." This phase may be nine years, nine months, nine weeks, or even nine days. This concept can be further extended to nine milliseconds on the one hand and nine lifetimes on the other.

Mudras, Divine Communication

One of the main features of the Gitananda tradition is the detailed exposition and understanding of Mudra, the ancient Yogic art and science of gesturing and sealing vital Prana. These advanced techniques are designed to improve neuromuscular coordination, refine human emotions, and still the restless mind. They enable us to communicate intrapersonally with our Inner Self, interpersonally with others, and transpersonally with the Divine. The teachings of Hasta Mudras (hasta mudrā) in the Vibhaga and Pranava Pranayamas (praṇava prāṇāyāma) highlighted in this book are unique to this tradition.

Create Gurus, not Followers

Pujya Swamiji never desired huge numbers of students, a multitude of ashrams, fame, or a vast organizational empire. All that mattered to him was the growth of the student, and he aimed to help manifest students' inherent potential even though this often meant being an exacting taskmaster. Each and every one of Swamiji's students became "the best" they could have been in this lifetime.

How This Book Came to Life

The teachings of Nada Yoga are an integral part of Rishiculture Ashtanga Yoga in the Parampara of Swami Gitananda Giri. Nada (nāda) is a Sanskrit term whose translation can be summarized as "vibration and sound," and which refers to those teachings in Gitananda Yoga that focus on the awareness, perception, and production of vibration, sound, and music. Gitananda Nada Yoga[2] principles and practices are integral to Rishiculture Ashtanga Yoga, not separate from it. These teachings have their roots in the two lineages of the Parampara—the Bengali Tantric Tradition and the Tamilian Shaiva Siddhanta—and, with Yogamaharishi Dr. Swami Gitananda Giri, they were also infused with Western medical language and reference systems. Yogacharya Dr. Ananda Balayogi Bhavanani has been continuing the tireless work of maintaining the authenticity of the teachings while keeping them relevant in medical, artistic, and spiritual contemporary circles for the benefit of all. "Sharing is caring" is one of Dr. Ananda's mottos, and this book is the result of such generosity of spirit and action.

In 2009, Yogacharini Dr. Sangeeta Laura Biagi began her studies of Rishiculture Ashtanga Yoga. Living in New York, where she was a college professor, Dr. Sangeeta enrolled in the *Yoga: Step-by-Step* course and, the following year, moved to Ananda Ashram in India to complete a six-month Yoga teacher training. While in residence at the Ashram, Sangeeta began her in-depth studies and practice of Nada Yoga under the direct guidance of Dr. Ananda and also began her studies of the traditional arts of Sanatana Dharma, in particular the classical form of Carnatic singing and Bharatanatyam dance with Yogacharini Devasena Bhavanani. Sangeeta lived in the Ashram for two years and then decided to come back to the United States and Europe to share these teachings.

During the pandemic of COVID-19, Dr. Ananda began sharing the teachings of Gitananda Yoga online, creating videos on various principles of Tantra, Yantra, and Mantra, as well as sharing live feeds of ritual celebrations

2 It is important to know that Swami Gitananda did not call his teachings on Nada "Gitananda Nada Yoga" and that it was Yogacharya Dr. Ananda Balayogi Bhavanani, his son and successor, and Yogacharini Dr. Sangeeta Laura Biagi, their student, who coined this title to create online and in-person training programs beginning in 2021.

taking place at the Ashram and at the Gurus' Samadhi site, Sri Kambaliswami Madam. Dr. Ananda also converted various forms of training, which were previously held in person or by postal correspondence, to online training programs in which Dr. Sangeeta participated as a student and, sometimes, as a Mentor to other students. In the summer of 2021, Dr. Ananda invited Dr. Sangeeta to co-create an online course focusing on the teachings of the Parampara on Nada Yoga, which resulted in an online seven-month Nada Yoga immersion that was held once a week from December 2021 until June 2022, and which saw the participation of over 70 students from around the world. This course was followed by another online immersion, *Sacred Sounds of the Chakras*, in November and December 2022, and a residential intensive course at Ananda Ashram on March 2–16, 2023.

While teaching these courses, Dr. Sangeeta and Dr. Ananda made the decision to share the teachings in a book format and the choice of collaborating with Singing Dragon solidified. The process of choosing which principles and practices to share and how to make them accessible in writing—considering that all teachings rely on oral transmission—was often challenging and required awareness of the format's limitations and strengths. Given the width and depth of the teachings of Rishiculture Ashtanga Yoga, this book is designed to be an introduction to the wealth of the principles and practices of the Gitananda Parampara, with the hope of inspiring readers to take in-depth studies (online and in person) to become, themselves, capable of sharing them with authenticity and respect.

Chapter 1 is an introduction to Nada Yoga and the meaning and applications of its philosophy in our day-to-day life. In particular, the authors focus on the importance of learning how listening and sound vibrations affect our various bodies (pañca kośa) and how a conscious invocation of sound in the form of Mantra may contribute to our overall health.

Chapter 2 focuses on the Mantra of Mantras, the Pranava Om (praṇava oṃ). This Mantra has been praised for millennia as the vibration of the Divine incarnate. In this chapter, the authors will share Swami Gitananda's system of sectional breathing practices, the Vibhaga Pranayama, which employs the use of the hands in various gestures called Hasta Mudras to stimulate various parts of the lungs and create reflexogenic flows from the fingertips to our breathing center in the medulla oblongata of the brainstem. The relationship between breathing, listening, and vocal invocation of the Mantra is at the heart of the Pranava Pranayama, a real gem of this Parampara.

Chapter 3 offers an overview of the complex system of psychic energies called Chakras. The authors introduce the six lower and six higher energy centers, focusing on the lower six, the Pinda Chakras (piṇḍa cakra), and their correspondences in the cerebrospinal human system and their "seed sounds," the Bija Mantras as well as the Devata Gayatri Mantras (devatā gāyatrī mantra) for each of the Shat Chakras (ṣaṭ cakra).

Chapter 4 introduces some fundamental concepts of Yoga Chikitsa (yoga cikitsā), Yoga Therapy, and how the principles and practices of Gitananda Nada Yoga offer excellent tools to generate and maintain physical, emotional, mental, and spiritual health.

Appendix I offers a selection of Mantras we invoke in our daily practices (sādhana) at Ananda Ashram. Appendix II highlights some of the research studies conducted at the Institute of Salutogenesis and Complementary Medicine of the Sri Balaji Vidyapeeth (Deemed-to-Be University) by Dr. Ananda and colleagues at the Institute's School for Yoga Therapy and School for Music Therapy previously known as the CYTER and CMTER. Appendix III contains a selection of entries written by members of the Gitananda Nada Yoga community worldwide. Their writings were collected in the form of weekly assignments during the seven-month online Nada Yoga course that Dr. Ananda and Dr. Sangeeta taught between December 2021 and June 2022.

Chapter I

NADA YOGA

The Sound of Yoga is Silence[1]

Nada is a pure vibration that is eternal: it has always existed, is always existing, and will always exist because it is the vibrational essence of the Universe. The Sanskrit term Nada expresses the quality of a "vibratory flow," an expression of the life force, and an instrument to inquire into the nature of reality. This pure vibration is so subtle that it emanates at the level of the causal body, the Karana (kāraṇa) Sharira (śarīra), also known as the astral body, the Linga (liṅga) Sharira. It is complex to describe this frequency of vibration because Nada is "without form" (arūpa) and "without name" (anāmi), and it has no material qualifications (nirguṇa), existing "beyond the gunas" (guṇa), the qualities of nature, and the mind. More than a quantitative substance, Nada is a qualitative essence.

Nada Yoga is often translated as the "Yoga of Sound." However, "expressed sound" is best defined as Shabda (śabda), a term referring to that which is heard by the auditory apparatus and interpreted as noise, environmental sounds, music, or language. Nada Yoga may be defined as the theoretical and analytical understanding of the universal primordial vibration, coupled with a dedicated practice of sounds at different levels of being for the purpose of attaining universal Oneness. While Shabda can be perceived through our senses, including the sixth sense of the mind (manas), Nada may only be perceived in the Silence of the Heart (hṛdaya). This is the "psychic heart" of Anahata Chakra (anāhata chakra), the "wheel of energy" of "unstruck sound." Why is silence perceived here, in the area that physically and physiologically corresponds to our heart, which pumps and beats from

1 This is a teaching that is very dear to Ammaji Yogacharini Meenakshi Devi Bhavanani.

the day we are born to the day we die, and which corresponds also to our lungs, that receive and expel air from the day we are born until the day we die? What is the relationship between the sound of our heart pumping, our breath flowing, and the silence of their higher psychic vibration?

The silence of causal vibration is the Anahata Nada (anāhata nāda), the "unstruck sound" that exists before a cause and is, therefore, causal. It is not an absence of sound; rather, it is the absorption of mind in the vibratory essence of reality. This reabsorption (laya) is achieved in a step-by-step system of practice (sādhana) that relies on a conscious and gradual refinement of our senses, particularly our sense of hearing, and of how we relate to sound, including the sound of our voice and the way we think and utter sound. Awareness of the perception of outer and inner sounds transforms the physiological sense of hearing into conscious listening, a precious tool to gain self-knowledge.

When left unattended, the subconscious mind creates a field of noise that clouds our capacity to experience unity with life. The untamed flow of memories from the past and projections for the future build a matrix of vibrations that keep us distracted from what is occurring here and now, in the present moment. In the first Pada (pāda) of the *Yoga Sutra*,[2] second aphorism, Maharishi Patanjali teaches us that Yoga is the quieting of such noise:

> [I:2]
>
> योगश्चित्तवृत्तिनिरोधः ॥२॥
>
> yogaścittavṛttinirodhaḥ
>
> *Yoga is the cessation of the whirlpools of the subconscious mind* (Bhavanani, 2011a, p.33).

As Dr. Ananda explains:

> Whenever the conscious mind tries to deal with the subconscious mind, we are sucked under—this is why Swami Gitananda explains the Cittavritti as the "whirlpools of the subconscious mind." Before we know it, we are pulled

2 The *Yoga Sutras* are a composition of 196 aphorisms (sūtra) that, in a step-by-step manner, instruct the seeker on the principles and practices of the Yoga Darshana, a reverential view of the highest reality through the art and science of Yoga. Transmitted in an oral form, the written *Sutras* are dated to a period between the 4th century BCE and the 3rd century CE.

> down to the bottom of the ocean. The process of yoga is the method of bringing these subconscious and unconscious activities up to the conscious level. (Bhavanani, 2011a, p.33)

Thanks to continued practice, a blend of effort and "dispassionate detachment," the internal noise subdues and deeper aspects of Nada Yoga reveal themselves. Maharishi Patanjali names these two Abyhasa and Vairagya (vairāgya):

> [I:12]
>
> अभ्यासवैराग्याभ्यां तन्निरोधः ॥
>
> abhyāsavairāgyābhyāṃ tannirōdhaḥ
>
> *Their* [of the Citta Vrittis] *cessation is brought about by effort coupled with objectivity* (Bhavanani, 2011a, p.48).

Step by step, Sadhakas, Seekers of Truth (sādhaka), learn to outgrow the "obstacles" on the Yoga path, what Maharishi Patanjali describes as the Pancha Klesha (pañca kleśa), the most challenging of which is "attachment to life and fear of death," the survival instinct of Abhinivesha (abhiniveśa) [II:3]. There is a primal connection between the noise of the Citta Vritti (cittavṛtti) and Abhinivesha Klesha, and we all are called to reflect on how this manifests in our lives. Swami Gitananda used to say that most people suffer from "verbal diarrhea" and, while the image may be a bit shocking at first, we soon realize this is the truth. Most people fill their lives with noise, so they do not think about, let alone prepare for, their death. Death is part of life and Yoga Sadhana is a healthy and happy preparation for this sacred moment in our lives. When we are able to overcome the "horror vacui," the terror of the void that we fear exists beyond noise, we can fully relax.

In Gitananda Nada Yoga, the voice, which for most people, including Yoga practitioners and teachers, is fairly unknown territory, is cultured through the understanding and practice of the Sanskrit phonemes as manifesting from the immortal sound of the Pranava AUM in the articulation of the Bija Mantras, sacred seed sounds, and their combination in longer Mantras, such as the Panchakshara Mantra (pañcākṣara mantra) Om Namah Shivaya (oṁ namaḥ śivāya), a salutation to Lord Shiva (śiva) which contains the five syllables (akṣara) "Na," "Ma," "Shi," "Va," "Ya." This Parampara also offers a repertoire of devotional chants, the Bhajans (bhajan),[3] and a study of classical Carnatic music which supports a Sadhana aimed at sensorial refinement, self-control, and self-knowledge. All of these "sound practices" are a means to gain mental equipoise by focusing the mind and, via "entrainment,"[4] quiet inner and outer vibratory disturbances. The result is a blissful state of calm and serenity that may be experienced for a few seconds at first, then prolonged to a few minutes, and, with the grace of the Guru (guru),[5] held for an uninterrupted flow as an integral part of our everyday life.

The cultivation of inner and outer silence, Mauna (mauna), is at the heart of the teachings of Gitananda Yoga. As Swamiji's Dharmapatni (dharmapatnī, wife and spiritual companion), Puduvai Shakti Puduvai Kalaimamani Yogacharini Meenakshi Devi Bhavanani, henceforth referred to as Pujya Ammaji, teaches us, "The Sound of Yoga is Silence." One of the aspects of the great Lord Shiva, the "God of Yoga" (yogeśvara = yoga īśvara), is Dakshina Murti (dakṣiṇā mūrti), "the form of the divine teacher who sits in the north facing south," the direction that is associated with the deity presiding death, Lord Yama (yama). Sri Adi Shankaracharya (Śaṅkarācārya), the 8th century CE philosopher and theologian of Advaita Vedanta (advaitavedānta), in the *Dakshina Murti Stotra* (dakṣiṇamūrti stotra), a spiritual and religious hymn in praise of Lord Shiva, describes the Lord as Mauna Vakya (mauna vākya), a teacher who teaches through this state of inner and outer silence which contains all sonic vibrations, just like white light contains all the vibrations of the color spectrum.

The Journey of Vibrations: Nada, Bindu, Kala

The system of cosmogony that supports the understanding of a process of reabsorption into an original cosmic vibration is not that different from the astronomical theory of a Big Bang. Developed in 1927 by astronomer

---

3 A selection of Bhajans is shared in Appendix I.

4 In physics and biology, entrainment signifies a phenomenon of sympathetic resonance through which something is made to have the same pattern or rhythm as something else. It is used in music and sound studies to describe how a prayer or, in this case, a Mantra is able to regulate the waves of thought by absorbing them into its resonance.

5 Guru is a Sanskrit term that refers to a "dispeller of the darkness of ignorance" ("gu," darkness, and "ru," dispeller). The word Guru refers to an energetic force that dwells inside the psychic heart of each person. It also refers to an enlightened being who is One with the essence of All that Is and who can help others attain that state.

Georges Lemaître, the theory explains that the universe began from a single point and then, over 13.8 billion years, stretched and expanded to its current dimensions. Two years later, Edwin Hubble noticed that other galaxies were moving away from our solar system and that the furthest galaxies from us were moving faster than the ones close to us, implying that the universe is still expanding.[6] Astronomers are still debating what was there before that big first explosion or what originated it. What was there beyond that single point of origination?

Yoga teachings have been offering an answer since antiquity. Before manifestation, there existed a Cosmic Intelligence, called by as many names as there are traditions: Para-Brahman (parabrahman), Para-Nada (paranāda), Ishwava (īśvara), Para-Shiva (paraśiva), Maha-Shakti (mahāśakti). In the process of creation of the manifest Universe, the essence of Para-Nada coalesced into a Bindu, a point of utmost energy condensation. This point is not the origin of manifestation but, rather, an aperture, a luminescent drop, a portal that connects unmanifest with manifest realities. It is here that the manifestation of the Mother Goddess, Mahamayi (mahāmayi), or the One who creates Maya (mayā), occurs as Kala (kalā),[7] a Sanskrit term that describes "the drama of life" and also refers to the human concept of "time."[8]

In the image on the following page, the process of manifestation is illustrated as an hourglass in which at the top we see the cosmic vibration of Nada, which manifests through the single point of the Bindu (the dot) as Kala. If we were to imagine the process of reabsorption from the drama of life back to the original vibration, we could turn the hourglass upside down. All of our drives, desires, memories, stories, and projections would need to be slowly refined and reabsorbed to condense back into the Bindu to access the metaphysical experience of Samadhi in Nada.

As Shakespeare reminds us, "the world's a stage," and we are players mouthing our lines and spinning our stories. When the time is up, we go off the stage. To continue using a theater metaphor, once we are ready to leave our bodies, the "show" ends for us but not for the ones who are still in the theater, engaged with the play. Through Nada Yoga practices, we consciously

---

6 Sourced from the NASA educational website, NASA Space Place (2023).

7 Also called Mahashakti (mahāśakti) and Prakriti (the primary substance).

8 Kala is also used to refer to the dramatic arts of India as, for example, dance, which is called Natyakala (nāṭyakāla).

engage in a process of reabsorption (laya) "back" to the original vibration, Para-Nada, from the physical to the subtle (Kala-Bindu-Nada).

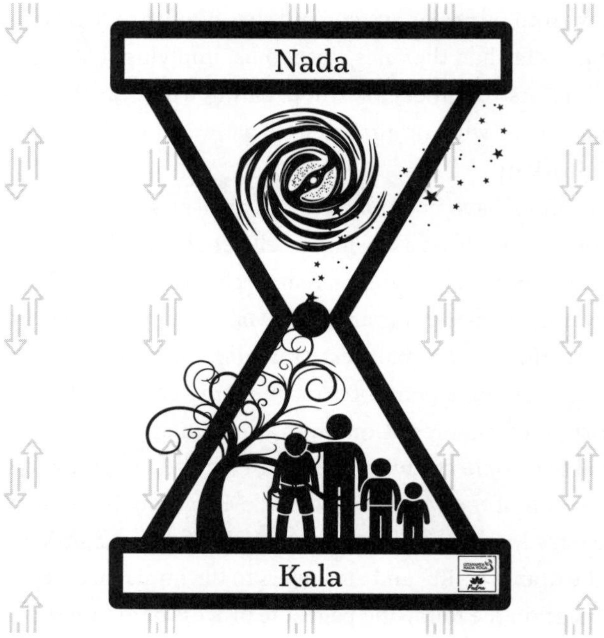

Nada, Bindu, Kala
A color version of this image can be downloaded from uk.singingdragon.com/catalogue/book/9781839974502.

Our conception and birth process follows this pattern as well: the seed energy of the sperm in the causal body, the Karana Sharira (kāraṇa śarīra), enters the ovum as a Bindu in the subtle body of the Sukshma (sūkṣma) Sharira to create human life in the gross body, the Sthula (sthūla) Sharira. When we are born, our experience of Kala begins manifesting as our personality. At the level of sound, our personality expresses itself through storytelling—the stories we slowly create about who we are in society (our name, family relations, social relations, fame, profession, and so on). Yoga, as a way of life, sustains our desire to live by the spiritual laws that guide our life (svadharma) to fully express our potential and contribute to our communities. While being in the world, however, we remember that everything is transitory. The desire to evolve through reabsorption, and the connected withdrawal from the pleasure of sensorial "drama," should not be confused as a denial of life, or a form of denigration of the senses. On the contrary, it is only by learning to live life fully, in a good and balanced way, that we understand the nature of reality.

Vibratory Five-Fold Awareness

Reality is a manifestation of the cosmic life energy of Nada. All sensations come into our body through transduction in various forms of vibrations. Our perception of smell, taste, sight, touch, hearing, and mentation is vibratory in nature. Everything that vibrates creates a sound. However, if the object vibrating is infinitesimally small, such as an atom, or exponentially distant, such as a sound sourced from afar, we can't hear it. We perceive colors within the light spectrum that our eyes can see or perceive sounds within the frequencies that our ears can hear. This is true for all our senses, including our mind, because we can only think thoughts within the limits of our life's experience and conditioning. Therefore, this is where our journey back "hOMe"[9] begins: within the limitations of our human terrestrial experience.

The science and art of Yoga teach us that we are equipped with the necessary instruments for this journey: we have our five "action senses," the Karmendriyas (karmendriya), and our five "cognitive senses," the Jnanendriyas (jñānendriya), through which we perceive the five subtle elements, the Tanmatras (tanmātrā), and the five gross elements, the Mahabhutas (mahābhūta). These are windows to experience Kala. Awareness of all these layers of sensory perception requires focus and patience. Yogamaharishi Dr. Swami Gitananda Giri, in Lesson Three of *Yoga: Step-by-Step*, reveals one of the pillars of Yoga Sadhana: "Four-Fold Awareness." These teachings apply to all aspects of Yoga, including our studies in Nada Yoga. Swamiji writes:

> Yoga is conscious evolution. There is the general evolution of life, outside of the realm of consciousness, but that evolution lies in Cosmic Hands. Your evolution rests in your own hands—and it must be conscious, through sensitive awareness. (Giri, 1976, p.9)

Awareness, in the teachings of Swamiji, has four stages. The first is "awareness of the body"—of how it works and what it does. The Four-Fold process

---

9 "hOMe"" is a play on words that Dr. Ananda uses when teaching about evolution and the journey of coming back to the source, which is the Mantra OM. Hence, hOMe highlights the OM within the word home.

always begins here, at the lowest speed of vibration of the physical physiological body. The human sense of hearing physical sound is accomplished by the process of auditory transduction. We receive sound waves in the tympanic membrane of our outer ear and, through the vibration of the ossicles in the middle ear, send signals to the fluid hair cells of the inner ear. Here, sound waves become electrical impulses that are sent to the auditory nerve and interpreted as "music," "sound," or "language." We also hear sounds by feeling their vibrations through our skin and as they resonate in our bone structure via bone conduction. In the practices of Nada Yoga, this involves a steady concentration on the perceivable sounds of our body, such as the inner sounds of our heart pumping, our breath flowing, and our mind thinking. Through the awareness of the body, we also learn how to refine our listening skills by becoming aware of the sounds in our environment, from the closest to the furthest ones.

The second stage is "awareness of the effect of the emotions upon the body" and how "right emotions have a positive, beneficial effect upon the body, and that negative, destructive emotions have a powerful detrimental effect upon the body" (Giri, 1976, p.9). Swamiji gives us a recommendation on how to gain control over the rush of emotions:

> Learn to be aware of your emotions as soon as the emotion arises. Be quickly aware before you are out of control. Give over only to the powerful positive emotions, resisting and controlling the negative. (Giri, 1976, p.9)

Our emotions influence the way we perceive sounds, make non-verbal sounds, or compose music. Even more importantly, emotions have a direct impact on the quality of our inhalation and exhalation. Anger, jealousy, malice, or greed result in specific types of breathing patterns such as unconscious held-in or held-out breaths, fast uncontrolled breaths, and so on. Learning to control the breath, by listening to it, is a great tool to refine our emotional intelligence. In Indian classical music, different Ragas (rāga), ways in which various tones are organized in an ascending and descending musical scale, stimulate particular Rasas (rasa), "flavors" or "moods" (Nagarajan, 2021).

The third stage is "awareness of the mind and how the mind can control the emotions and the body" (Giri, 1976, p.9). Swamiji offers a clear definition of the aspects of the mind:

> ADHI-VYADHI [ādhi-vyādhi] is the Sanskrit term suggesting the higher mind, the conscious mind. ADHI-VYADHI is our term for psycho-somatics. When this phase is accomplished, a new awareness can be sought, one in which the conscious mind is transcended by a higher aspect of the mind called the Buddhi. Chitta is sub-consciousness. Manas is consciousness. The Buddhi is the higher faculty of awareness, sometimes dubbed the intellect. Dharana, concentration, and Dhyana, meditation, are used to produce this awareness. (Giri, 1976, p.9)

The practices of Mantra Yoga, an integral part of Nada Yoga, help us gain control over all these aspects of the mind by tuning in to the mind's sub-conscious vibrations, the Citta Vritti, quieting them through the power of a conscious use of Mantra and elevating them to subtler vibrations of Nada.

The fourth stage is "awareness of awareness itself." Swamiji defines this stage as "Samadhi or Cosmic Consciousness." This is the state of Oneness with Para-Nada, a complete absorption into the vibration of Self, in which the individual self ceases to be differentiated and therefore subject to the laws of time and space. Ammaji added a fifth stage, "the awareness of how unaware we are." This, in fact, is more like a preliminary stage or a stage that applies to all others. We always need to remind ourselves to "stay aware" or, as Ammaji teaches us, "remember to remember" or, in this context, remember to listen. Listen to inner sounds, outer sounds, the sound of thoughts, Divine sounds in nature: life is a symphony! As an old saying goes, "Beauty is in the eye of the beholder." We may chime in, "Harmony is in the heart of the listener."

The Four Levels of Nada and the Power of Nama-Rupa

According to traditional Yoga teachings, there are three levels of Nada, differentiated by the refinement of their vibratory states from the grossest to the subtlest:

- Vaikhari (vaikharī): expressed language that others can hear and understand
- Madhyama (madhyama): awareness of sound in one's mind
- Pashyanti (paśayanti): the condensation of Nada and a subtle intuition of its energy.

Beyond these, and encompassing them, there is a most subtle state of Supreme Vibration, the Para-Nada (paranāda), which is transcendental and beyond our sensorial perception.

When we intone a Mantra, we operate at the level of Vaikhari Nada. When we think or contemplate a sound, we operate at the level of Madhyama Nada. These uttered and mentally formulated sounds set up a ripple effect into the Pashyanti and Para-Nada levels of frequency, too. Through the Nada Yoga practices, we create, internally and externally, new healthy patterns, Sankalpas (saṅkalpa), which create positive impressions, and Samskaras (saṃskāra), which replace the destructive energy of negative thinking and speech. We need to use our intellect, the Buddhi (buddhi), to consciously invoke the reality we want to manifest and live in.

The vibrational essence of that "thing" is its name (nāma), which we can cognize, write, and express. Nama is not a label or just a name: it is an invocation. Whatever we invoke by name, we evoke by manifestation, Rupa (rūpa). Nama and Rupa are one. In Sanskrit, each sound is a coded version of the energy we invoke, like a password that opens us up to the treasure that lies within or like the sign or number in a mathematical formula. Evoking, the other aspect of our practices, is to manifest: we evoke that which we invoke. This is one of the reasons why it is so important to maintain the Sanskrit names for Yogic teachings, as they contain the essence, Sara (sāra), of concepts, ideas, and teachings. Sanskrit is a comprehensive language that stimulates our whole vocal apparatus. Vowels and consonants, in their articulation of guttural, palatal, dental, labial, nasal, and cerebral sounds, are created by the specific movement of the muscles of our oral cavity, especially the positioning and shape of the tongue. The comprehensive vibratory essence of Sanskrit also manifests in the one-to-one correlation between the 50 Sanskrit phonemes with the 50 energetic "petals" of the Pinda Chakras, the energy centers located along the cerebrospinal axis.

In ancient times, the Rishis, wise men and women of India (sanātana dharma, the lands of the "eternal spiritual laws"), were able to attune themselves to the vibratory essence of Nada as a result of their disciplined efforts (tapasyā) in self-knowledge. The pure intellectual forms and sounds of the Sanskrit alphabet, the varṇamālā, the sacred garland of letters, revealed themselves to the Rishis who "heard" them (śruti)[10] in deep meditation and

10 Shruti is also a term used to describe the tonal note of Carnatic music.

then uttered them in the closest oral human approximation possible. Mantras (mantra) came into being as a result of their clairvision and clairaudience and so did the ancient *Vedas*,[11] composed in Vedic Sanskrit, which are defined as Apurusheyam (apuruṣeyam), "not made by men," and Anaadi (anādi), "without beginning" (Saraswati, 2009, p.3). These formulas and mantras were passed down orally through complex mnemonic systems before they were written down in books. Even today, a Mantra that is invoked mentally or orally is considered to be more powerful than a written text.

The Yoga Darshana (yoga darśana) is one of the six philosophies of Sanatana Dharma (sanātana dharma),[12] a living tradition best transmitted and learned orally, directly from the mouth of a Guru to the ears of the disciples. Oral teachings have been passed down from generation to generation, and therefore, great importance is given to the capacity to listen to the teachings, contemplate them, and make them true in one's life. In Yoga, there are the three levels of learning, each one based in the establishment of the previous:

- Shravana (śravaṇa): listening to the teachings of the Guru and allowing them to resonate in one's ears and heart
- Manana (manana): mentally understanding the concepts by contemplating them
- Nididhyasana (nididhyāsana): becoming one with the teachings by fully living the teachings and embodying them.

The "voice" of the Guru, the physiological voice as well as the vibration of the Guru's spirit, is a guiding force in one's practice. At Ananda Ashram, vocal sounds fill the halls and rooms. Those who met Swamiji in person take great pleasure in remembering his booming voice when he taught or when he burst into song or laughter. The same is true for Ammaji, Dr.

---

11 The four *Vedas* are: *Rigveda*, a collection of Vedic Sanskrit hymns and Mantras composed of verses (ric); the *Yajurveda* (yajurveda), a collection of Mantras for specific religious rites (yajur); the *Samaveda* (sāmaveda), a collection of songs and melodies, the sāmans, from which the classical Indian styles of music, chanted for offerings and sacrifice, were developed; the *Atharvaveda*, a collection of Mantras invoked during ceremonies such as birth, marriage, and death, and used to invoke benevolent energies and counteract Karmic bondage.

12 In Hindu philosophy, the Shat Darshanas (ṣaṭ darśana) are six "views" on reality, existential philosophies applied to all aspects of living: Samkhya (sāṃkhya), Yoga, Nyaya (nyāya), Vaisheshika (vaiśeṣika), Mimamsa (mīmāṃsā), and Vedanta (vedānta).

Ananda, and the other members of the Bhavanani and Gitananda family. The capacity to express one's voice, physically and metaphorically, is integral to the teachings of this lineage. The vocal practice of Sanskrit, Carnatic music, Bhajans, and Mantra is essential in our training programs. This is not just a matter of predisposition. Rather, it is a Tantric teaching on the divinity of the voice.

Vac

The word "voice" came to English from the Latin "vox" and can be traced back to the Vedic Sanskrit term Vac (vāk), a Vedic ancestral divinity who symbolizes both the Cosmic vibratory principle of Nada and the process of its manifestation into Prakriti (prakṛti), the consensual reality we live in.[13] Vac is a feminine principle, a Shakti (śakti), fertile and receptive, a Divine Mother (mātṛka) that appears as early as the *Rigveda* (ṛgveda). Vac corresponds to "The Word" of the *Old Testament* and is both the originating vibration and its uttered manifestation. Later, Vac came to be understood as a faculty of the mind and, with attributes, she may also be portrayed as the goddess of knowledge, learning, music, and language, Shree Saraswati (Sarasvatī), the consort of Brahma, holding the four *Vedas* in her left lower hand. Saraswati also holds the Vina (vīṇā), a string instrument typical of classical Carnatic music, a symbol of our vertebral column and the subtle energy channel of Sushumna Nadi (suṣumṇā nadī). The sound of the Vina, as we will see later in this chapter, is also one of the Dasha Dhun (daśa dhun), the ten inner sounds felt in the body during meditation on Nada.

Our voice is, therefore, not a mere instrument to express our thoughts in verbal language or emotions in non-verbal language. The voice, to be precise, is not even "ours." It is the manifestation of Vac, the energy to create specific sounds that may bring us as close as possible to the causal vibration of Nada. Hence, how we understand and employ the voice is of the greatest importance. It took humans millions of years to evolve into two-legged mammals who stand up. In the process, our larynx lengthened and the muscles of the neck and throat refined to the extent that we are able to control the stretching of the vocal cords in very precise movements

13 Many of the verbs and adjectives we use in our Nada Yoga principles and practices derive from the word Vac, such as, for example, "in-voke," "e-voke," "voc-ation," "voc-alization."

that create the articulation of idioms. It is inspiring to observe the vocal cords in motion. We recommend you find videos of laryngoscopies on the internet to witness and better understand the vibration of the vocal cords in the utterance of sound. They look like a portal whose doors open and close, in a wave-like motion, thanks to the airflow.

The voice box, and the neck in general, is a very important area of our body. It is in this area that nerves that are vital to our survival and overall sensory perception innervate, such as the vagus nerve in the brainstem, the phrenic nerves in the cervical area of C3 to C5, and the trigeminal nerve in the area of cervical C5. Our throat is a funnel through which we inhale and exhale air, food, and fluids, and our ear canal is connected to the throat via the Eustachian tubes, making the ears and the throat an intimate pair. This is also one of the most delicate areas of the body. The spinal vertebrae at this region, the cervical vertebrae, are the smallest of the spine, and the muscles of the neck are also quite small in relation to other muscles in the body. Why have humans evolved in a way that one of the most delicate areas is also one of the most vital?

From a physical point of view, this can be explained by reflecting on the flexibility of the neck region. We are able to turn our heads in a great spectrum of angles to provide vision and hearing. We are able to control the movements of the chin, to rotate left and right, up and down, and diagonally, and to turn the head without moving the shoulders. When engaging the shoulders, and without moving the base of our torso or legs, we can look straight behind us. From an energetic and spiritual point of view, however, the shape of the neck makes even more sense. The neck is a portal and a bridge between the mind, Ajna Chakra (ajña cakra), and the heart, Anahata Chakra. If we employ the image of the hourglass that we used earlier to describe the evolutionary process of manifestation of Nada-Bindu-Kala, the vocal cords may be understood as the Bindu, the energetic point where the subtle vibration of Para-Vac (parā vāk) materializes as Vaikhari Vac (vaikharī vāk).

Inner Sounds

In Lesson Four of *Yoga: Step-by-Step*, Swami Gitananda wrote:

> it is not really too soon to start talking about inner experience of Awareness

> and meditation, although it may be a long time before we can actually understand what meditation really is. The early experiences of Dhyana, Yoga meditation, are those with a profound sense of lightness and joy. The joy is referred to in Sanskrit as "Anandam." The light is real light, triggered off within a hollow stem of a section of the nervous system and is called Murdhani Jyoti. There is a counterpart to this "Light generated within the nervous system" that is termed "Cosmic Light." Whatever the source of the light, one can undertake a beautiful restful, inner gaze on this Inner Light. Learn to gaze into the light, and never grasp. The light will disappear if you try to possess it. Sometimes sound will arise from within. It may be simply inner body sounds, or it may be the authentic "Cosmic Chant." Mystics have termed the "Inner Sound" Antara Shabdham, the Dhuni, or more correctly, the Dasa Dhun, the Ten Inner Sounds. The first sound usually heard is something like static electricity, a rustling or shuffling sound. Other sounds are like a flute, drums, a conch shell blowing, bells ringing, and the clap of thunder. (Giri, 1976, p.14)

The teachings on the ten inner sounds, the Dasha Dhun or Dasa Dwani (daśa dhvani), are esoteric, and their realization requires a steady and disciplined practice. This commitment is meaningful, as the experience of inner sounds is blissful, beyond the quality of joy we experience when our sensual desires are fulfilled. In fact, it is an experience of joy that only the conscious withdrawal of desire can guarantee. "Never grasp," Swamiji warns us, because as soon as we desire to "be more and have more," joy, just like inner light, disappears. The practice of listening to the inner sounds abides by the same rules. If one is to search for the sounds, they will not manifest. The mind in the process of "craving" is too busy with gross thoughts to allow inner sounds to arise. The inner sounds are heard in a "meditative state of being," at the level of Pashyanti Vac, and cannot be perceived by the rational mind (Madhyama Vac, madhyama vāk) or the senses (Vaikhari Vac). They arise only in silence and, according to various schools and traditions, they are perceived through the inner space of the right ear, in the Sushumna Nadi, in the area of the "Third Eye," the Bruhmadya Bindu (bhrūmadya bindu), or other Antara Drishti (āntara dṛṣṭi), a point of inner gazing. Swami Gitananda lists these sounds as: "1. bell, 2. ocean, 3. elephant, 4. flute, 5. clouds, 6. bee, 7. dragon-fly, 8. conch, 9. drum and 10. lute" (Giri, 2008, p.42).

Classical Hatha Yoga (haṭha yoga) scriptures, such as the *Hatha Yoga Pradipika*,[14] teach that the experience of hearing the inner sounds occurs in a state of Dhyana, a deep listening meditation on Nada, Nada Anusandhana (nādānusandhāna), which precedes the Self-realization of Samadhi [4:66]. Swami Muktibodhananda writes:

> Anusandhana means 'exploration' or 'search.' The idea is to explore the sound in all dimensions and to follow the vibration from gross to subtle, from Vaikhari Vac to Para Vac. Each level of sound is joined and dependent upon the other. (Muktibodhananda, 1998, pp.556–558)

Among the ten inner sounds listed in the *Hatha Yoga Pradipika* are: twinkling sounds like bells [4:70]; kettledrum (bherīśabda) [4:73]; the sound of a drum (mardaladhvanih) [4:74]; the tinkling sound of the flute resonating like a vina (vainavah śabdah kvanadvīnākvano) [4:76]; the sound of the ocean, clouds, kettledrum, jharjhara drum, conch, gong, and horn [4:85]; the humming of bees [4:86]:

[4:85]

आदौ जलधि-जीमूत-भेरी-झर्झर-सम्भवाः ।
मध्ये मर्दल-शङ्खोत्था घण्टा-काहलजास्तथा ॥ ८५ ॥

ādau jaladhi-jīmūta-bherī-jharjhara-sambhavāḥ
madhye mardala-śaṅkhotthā ghaṇṭā-kāhalajāstathā

The first fruits are the sounds of the ocean, then clouds, the kettledrum and jharjhara drum. In the middle stage the shankha (conch), gong and horn (Muktibodhananda, 1998, p.581).

[4:86]

अन्ते तु किङ्किणी-वंश-वीणा-भ्रमर-निःस्वनाः ।
इति नानाविधा नादाः श्रूयन्ते देह-मध्यगाः ॥८६॥

14 The *Hatha Yoga Pradipika* is a classic text of Hatha Yoga, compiled by Svātmārāma in the 15th century CE in India. In its four chapters, a selection of classic Asanas (Chapter 1), Pranayamas (Chapter 2), and Mudras (Chapter 3) are described in a step-by-step manner to attain a state of union, Samadhi. While the teachings offer complete practices, enriched with the description of when, how, and why one should practice, there is a level of secrecy that veils and preserves their deepest layer. These are teachings for Sadhakas, practitioners who have already been studying under the guidance of a true Guru.

ante tu kingkiṇī-vaṃśa-vīṇā-bhramara-niḥsvanāḥ
iti nānāvidhā nādāḥ śrūyante deha-madhyaghāḥ

Now, reaching the inner point of conclusion, are the tinkling of bells, flute, vina and humming of bees. Thus, the various nadas are produced and heard from the middle of the body (Muktibodhananda, 1998, p.581).

Verses 88 and 89 warn the Sadhaka that, despite the great variety of sounds, Dharana is held on the subtlest of vibrations without getting distracted. Verse 90 offers a poetic simile:

[4:90]

मकरन्दं पिबन् भृङ्गी गन्धं नापेक्षते यथा ।
नादासक्तं तथा चित्तं विषयान् नहि काङ्क्षते ॥९०॥

makarandaṃ piban bhṛṅgī gandhaṃ nāpekṣate yathā
nādāsaktaṃ tathā cittaṃ viṣayān nahi kāṅkṣate

Just as a bee drinking honey is unconcerned about the fragrance, so the mind engaged in nada is not craving for sensual objects (Muktibodhananda, 1998, p.581).

Beyond these subtle sounds, when the Yogi has reached a state of complete stillness (unmanī), is silence. Silence, as the vibrant sound of Samadhi, is a peak experience of Raja Yoga, the royal path of victory over Death [103]. The senses are so subtle that even the subtlest of sounds, the ones of the conch (śangkha) or the Dundhubi drum (dundhubhi-nādaṃ), won't be heard anymore [106]. This is the Samadhi state of being, beyond the effects of time and karma (kālena bādhyate na ca karmaṇā) [108], a state of pure resonance where one cannot be killed because it is beyond the construction of death and is not even subject to the powerful laws of sacred geometry that sustain the manifest Universe Yantra, and their utterance, Mantra (mantra-yantrāṇāṃ) [113].

The *Gheranda Samhita* (Gheraṇḍa Saṃhitā) is another classical scripture of Hatha Yoga, a "Tantrika work" consisting of a dialogue between the sage Gheranda and the Sadhaka Chandakapali (Caṇḍakāpāli).[15] The book, dated

15 A question was raised by our esteemed colleague Yogacharya Bharata Bill Francis Barry on the problem of verse number differences in different translations of the *Gheranda Samhita*. In this book, we chose the following edition: *Gheraṇḍa Saṃhitā*, edited by Swami Digambarji and Dr. M.L. Gharote (1997).

around the 16th century CE, is divided into seven parts and contains over 350 verses. Part 5 is dedicated to Pranayama, the conscious control of the life force of Prana[16] through breathing patterns. In the section on the "Bee Sonic Breath," Bhramari Pranayama (bhramarī prāṇāyāma), the ten inner sounds are heard by listening "by the right ear," and they are:

[5:74–75]

मेघझर्झरभ्रमरी घण्टाकांस्यं ततः परम् ।
तुरीभेरीमृदङ्गादिनिनादानकदुन्दुभिः ॥ ७५ ॥

meghajharjharabhramarī ghaṇṭākāṃsyaṃ tataḥ param
turībherīmṛdaṅgādininādānakadundubhiḥ

sounds of cricket, flute, thunder, cymbals, big bee, bell, gong, trumpet, one sided drum, double sided drum[17] *in the order* (Digambarji and Gharote, 1997, p.137).

While some of the sounds differ from tradition to tradition, they all share a resonance that is full of harmonics—frequencies of pitches that vibrate in integer multiples of the fundamental frequency, which can be the drone of the bee, the fundamental note of the trumpet or the Vina, the percussive hit on a drum's skin, and, of course, the human voice, embodiment of Vak.

Medical studies confirm that the humming of our voice, when sustained for at least five minutes with a serene and relaxed attitude, produces excellent results in increasing our sense of health and well-being. This is because nasal and cerebral sounds stimulate the pituitary and pineal glands resulting in an increased production of nitric oxide, a molecule that is produced naturally by the body and whose most important function is vasodilation, allowing blood, nutrients, and oxygen to travel to every part of the body effectively and efficiently (a limited capacity to produce nitric oxide is associated with heart disease, diabetes, and erectile dysfunction) (Weitzberg and Lundberg, 2002, pp.144–145). Humming also increases the production of serotonin and dopamine, two "feel-good hormones." Serotonin, a neurotransmitter,

---

16 Prana, the "cosmic glue" that generates and sustains life as we know it and that we, as humans, perceive best through the awareness and regulation of breathing (prāṇāyāma) and through the nourishment of sun rays, food, and water. Prana is a vital life energy that we mostly perceive and absorb through breathing. Swami Gitananda defines Prana as "the Divine Mother Energy" and "the Universal Creative Power" (Giri, 1976, p.2).

17 Like a mṛdaṅga drum.

plays a major role in mood regulation. Dopamine is a neurotransmitter that is commonly associated with reward-motivated behavior and social anxiety. A research experiment found out that people with generalized social phobia tended to have lower dopamine levels than healthy subjects (Krishnakumar *et al.*, 2015, pp.13–19).

"Feeling good" and being well (well-being) are important reasons to embrace Nada Yoga Sadhana and very much in line with Swami Gitananda's teaching, "health and happiness are your birthright." The proliferation of New Age "sound healing" practices (sound massages, gong baths, tuning bowl concerts) is an indication of the level of the need for relaxation and ease. It is our responsibility to search for authentic teachings and practices that are rooted in medical study whether it be allopathic medicine, ayurvedic medicine, or indigenous medicine and inspired by spiritual wisdom so that we understand that meditation may entail the physiological effects of a "hormone shower" but that it is also a deeper process that requires practice and commitment towards self-awareness and refinement.

Prerequisites for Concentration (Dharana), Meditation (Dhyana), and Absorption (Samadhi)

Entering the word "meditation" on Google creates 740,000,000 results.[18] However, of these millions of people, only a few really understand the meaning of the word in the context of the sacred arts and sciences of Yoga. Meditation is a high vibrational state of conscious "mind-less-ness," rather than mind-full-ness, in the sense that, in meditation, there is "no mind" and no "thinking self." What most people refer to as meditation is, in fact, a form of concentration, Dharana, in which the person is able to remain aware of their posture, breathing, and thinking patterns for an extended period of time. Maharishi Patanjali commences the third part of the *Yoga Sutra*, Vibhuti Pada (vibhūti pāda), with one *Sutra* on Dharana:

[III:1]

देशबन्धश्चित्तस्य धारणा ॥ १ ॥

deśa-bandhaḥ cittasya dhāraṇā

---

18 In a Google search by the authors on February 18, 2023.

Binding our mind to one place is concentration
(Bhavanani, 2011a, p.217).

Dharana, Dr. Ananda explains, is "the exercise of consciousness, a process of awareness by which the entire mental apparatus is bound to or confined within a place, a point or a thing" (Bhavanani, 2011a, p.217). The *Sutras* continue with one aphorism on Dhyana, meditation:

[III.2]

तत्र प्रत्ययैकतानता ध्यानम् ॥ २ ॥

tatra pratyaya-ikatānatā dhyānam

Unbroken flow (of concentration) leads to meditative awareness (Bhavanani, 2011a, p.219).

Dr. Ananda comments:

> Dhyana implies an un-interrupted, continuous, unbroken, unwavering state of total attention. In the previous state of Dharana, there was a separate existence of object and subject. We, the subject, were concentrating on something, the object. In the state of meditation, however, subject and object have merged into one and are now one and the same. There is neither observer nor observed, but rather the state of observation. (Bhavanani, 2011a, p.219)

Dharana and Dhyana are preliminary steps to reach the state of beatitude of Samadhi:

[III.3]

तदेवार्थमात्रनिर्भासं स्वरूपशून्यमिव समाधिः ॥ ३ ॥

tadeva-artha-mātra-nirbhāsaṁ svarūpa-śūnyam-iva-samādhiḥ

Samadhi is the state wherein the essence alone remains without differentiation (Bhavanani, 2011a, p.222).

Samadhi is the culminating experience of Oneness. There is a quality of the mind, Sarvartha (sarvārtha), to describe a state in which we are unable to focus; in fact, we focus on too much (from artha, "things," and sarva, "everything"), which results in confusion and loss of direction in life. Dharana, Dhyana, and Samadhi constitute the progressive process of

Samyama (saṃyama), a "binding of the mind with the Absolute" in a unified form of "concentration—meditation—absorption" [III:4] that enables us to live in Prajna Loka (prājña loka), a state of Higher Consciousness. Samyama may be paralleled to the process of reabsorption, Laya, from a tantric perspective.

The highly refined progression of Sadhana is what the English translation of the scriptures describes as "meditation on the Anahata Nada," which most Yoga aspirants confuse with a concentration on sound. Once this has become clear, and equipped with courage and passion, the Yoga aspirants commit to becoming physically, emotionally, mentally, and spiritually "fit" thanks to the cultivated qualities of discipline, commitment, patience, faith, and, most importantly, a surrender to the Divine, a type of active relaxation that is rooted in fully trusting the wisdom of a Higher Cosmic Intelligence and of the teachings, as well as trusting one's efforts and sincerity.

In Rishiculture Ashtanga Yoga, following the teachings on Ashtanga Yoga, the Eightfold Royal Path codified by Maharishi Patanjali in the *Yoga Sutra* [II:29], we learn that as prerequisite to experiencing the uninterrupted flow of Samyama, we commit to the:

- study of and adherence to the Yamas and Niyamas, the five moral restraints and five ethical observances
- disciplined practice of Asana, physical, physiological, and energetic geometrical body postures
- disciplined practice of Pranayama, the conscious control of the life force of Prana through breathing patterns
- observance of Pratyahara (pratyāhāra): sensory refinement and withdrawal
- study and practice of specific Mudras (mudrā) such as: the Hasta Mudras performed in the lobular breathing of Vibhaga Pranayama and Pranava Pranayama;[19] the Shanmukhi Mudra (śanamukhī mudrā), a closing of the orifices of the face which accompanies Bhramari Pranayama; the Kechari Mudra (khecarī mudrā), a classical Yoga Mudra (yoga mudrā) in which the tip of the tongue is rolled back and

19 Detailed in Chapter 2.

placed in contact with the roof of the oral cavity, between the soft and hard palate, performed to create a humming cerebral sound in the invocation of Bija Mantras[20]

- adoption of a Yoga Bhavana (yoga bhāvana), a Yogic attitude to look for the good even in the unpleasant.

These, in fact, are only a few of the many steps we take in the journey of involution from our gross experience of reality to the inner subtle experience of Nada through the Samyama of concentration, meditation, and absorption.

Where to Start: Soham Mantra

When asked the question "Where to start?" Swamiji replied, "Where life starts... with the breath." The English word "breath" is derived from the Old English "bræð," which means "odor, scent, exhalation." In the 14th century CE this word gained the more current meaning of inhalation and exhalation, or a movement of air. In Latin, the word "spiritus" means "a respiration, the breath of life" from which the English verbs "in-spire" and "ex-pire" are derived, and from which the meaning of spirit as "angel, energy, ghost" also derived in the middle of the 14th century CE. Therefore, when we inhale and when we exhale, we "welcome the spirit" and allow ourselves to be "inspired" by its nourishing energy. These reflections find a correspondence in the Yoga teachings on Prana.

In the teachings of Yoga, and of Nada Yoga in particular, great importance is given to the sounds of our inhalation and exhalation. Breathing, as a movement of life energy (śakti), has its own specific sound. Our inhalations and exhalations are specific to us and, even though there is a general sense of what an inhale or an exhale sounds like, our breathing sonic patterns are specifically ours. Our breath, which is a vehicle for Prana to manifest at the gross material level, accompanies us from birth (our first inhalation) to death (our last exhalation). Each breath contains, in this sense, a lifetime of its own.

The Soham Mantra (soham mantra), also known as the Hamsa[21] Soham

20 Detailed in Chapter 3.

21 Hamsa, in Sanskrit, also refers to the white water swan, a bird that symbolizes purity, higher intellect, and learning, and an individual self that is attuned to the Divine Self. The swan is praised for its legendary ability to separate milk from water, a symbol of Viveka, "discernment," characteristic of those who walk sincerely on the Yoga path.

Mantra (haṃsaḥ soham mantra), is named the Ajapa Japa (ajapā japa) and Ajapa Gayatri (ajapā gāyatrī). The Soham Mantra is called the Ajapa Gayatri in the *Geranda Samhita* [5:79]: "[The breath] goes out making the sound Ham and comes in 21,600 times making the sound Sah during a day and night. This is called Ajapā Gāyatrī which every being repeats incessantly" (Digambarji and Gharote, 1997, p.138). Ajapa is the absence (a-) of uninterrupted invocation (japa), which means that the Mantra exists without a cause prior to the act of will implied in recitation. We have already found this negation in the word Anahata, which we translated as "unstruck" from the Sanskrit non (a-) percussed (ahata).

There is a connection between the vibratory essence of Anahata Nada and the manifestation of the Ajapa Japa in that they are both eternal and non-perishable. Even though the Ajapa Japa Mantra is often studied in relation to the cycles of human breathing (and is therefore perishable), its true vibration is of the realm of Ananda, eternal bliss, as the sound of the "Breath of God." "So" means "All that is/That" and "Ham" means "I am." "So" is the natural sound we make when we inhale, and "Ham" is the natural sound we make when we exhale. This is a subtle sound (ajapa) that already exists in us, and not a form of sonorous breathing style "we make." Concentration on these Mantric sounds happens at the level of non-uttered sound, Madhyama Vac.

"That, I am… I am That," an innate repetition that occurs 21,600 times each day. Our responsibility is to activate it with awareness and ignite it with focus. During the inhalation, we receive all of the nutrients in the surrounding atmosphere and beyond. As we inhale, we become "in-spired." Exhalation is connected to letting go of the carbon dioxide and the acidity in our blood, as well as the gift of sharing, because as we exhale, we offer our own unique selves to the world. Inhale, So, we receive; exhale, Ham, we share. We can begin with an even breath of 4x4 (4 inhale and 4 exhale) and then slowly extend the counts to 6x6 and higher. The goal is not the prolongation of the inhale and exhale. The goal is to reach a relaxed state of Kumbhaka (kumbhaka), a breath retention that is not an apnea but, rather, a natural cessation of the breath that does not result in, nor is the effect of, death. These are advanced practices that should not be attempted without the expert guide of a Guru or advanced teacher (ācārya).

To start, we can learn to control our senses, calm the mind's chitchat, and listen to the breath. This apparently simple practice is not that simple. The mind will soon become busy and will resist "silence." Pujya Ammaji describes the mind as a wild monkey on a hot rooftop, running here, there, and everywhere. However, once we are able to maintain the necessary Dharana for a few minutes, the ripple effect is immense and so refined that we may barely notice it at first. However, the health benefits are many. At the physiological-physical level, consciously regulating the breath and listening to its subtle sound slows our heart rate, lowers our blood pressure, and calms our thoughts. This activation of the parasympathetic nervous system allows us to feel a sense of ease and to gain control over negative emotions. The meaning of the Mantra reminds us that we are not alone, that we are part of something beautiful, that our lives matter, and that we are here for a Divine purpose. We chose to be here, on this planet, at this time. We embrace the responsibility of using our breath properly, of using the sound of our breath and the sound of our voice properly. We start to find that rhythm that lies within us, the rhythm of the Universe that manifests through us in our biorhythms. We harmonize and attune our inner rhythms physiologically, emotionally, mentally, and psychically with the Cosmos.

PRACTICE

1. Sit in a comfortable position on the floor or on a chair or lie down. Whatever you choose, make sure you are able to inhale and exhale freely. You may pick up a classical Asana such as Sukha Asana (sukha āsana), the "Pleasant Posture," sitting with your legs crossed, Vajra Asana (vajra āsana), the "Thunderbolt Posture," sitting with the glutei on your heels, or a more advanced Asana. If you are unable to sit on the floor, you may sit on a chair or lie down on a firm surface. It is important that your vertebral column and body are aligned to the best of your current capacity.

2. Inhale and exhale through the nostrils.

3. Scan your body to check whether you are holding unnecessary tension anywhere. Be meticulous in your process of "checking in" with yourself and make sure that the many muscles of your face (around the eyes, lips, and cheeks) and of your neck and shoulders are relaxed.

4. Relax your arms, hands, and fingers. Relax the entire area of the

torso—front, side, and back. Roll your shoulders back and down. Relax the muscles of the abdomen and the muscles of the upper, middle, and lower back. Relax your legs all the way to the feet and toes.

5. Begin to consciously deepen your breathing patterns. Make the inhale and the exhale even and regulate the breath on a specific count (such as 4x4 or 6x6). Witness what "comes up" as you regulate the breath. This is Sukha Pranayama (sukha prāṇāyāma).
6. When you feel established in this Pranayama, begin to listen deeply and inwardly to the sounds of the Ajapa Japa Mantra, Soham. "So" as you inhale, and "Ham" as you exhale.
7. Thoughts will arise and distract you. Come back to the Mantra Sadhana[22] (mantra sādhana) over and over again until you gain a feeling of being at ease with yourself and your inner and outer worlds.

How to Listen—Shabda Kriya and Shabda Pratyahara

Swami Gitananda, in Lesson Forty-Five of *Yoga: Step-by-Step*, teaches the practice of Shabda Pratyahara (śabda pratyāhara) (Giri, 1976, pp.211–212). This is a step-by-step process of concentration on the sounds inside our body, such as the heartbeat and the audible breath, and the sounds in our environment, from the closest to the furthest and then back to the closest. By contemplating sound from the grossest of vibrations to the subtlest, we retrace our journey from Sthula Sharira (sthūla śarīra), the manifested field of existence, to the Sukshma Sharira (sūkṣma śarīra), the subtle field of existence, and the Karana Sharira, the causal field of existence. In this form of Pratyahara we expand and refine our externalized senses before we consciously withdraw them inside of us, under the control of the mind, in an internalized para-sensory experience. Moving from a sensory experience based on sound to that of a para-sensory experience that is now based on vibration, we are moving from Kala, to Bindu, to Nada. The Shabda we hear becomes an object of contemplation. Our busy mind slowly relaxes and gets

22 Mantra Sadhana is the assiduous practice of Mantras.

absorbed in the essence of the Akasha Tattva (ākāśa tatva), the principle of space and ether, which offers the highest freedom of perception while we are in our physical bodies.

As Swamiji teaches us:

> be wise enough at this point to recognise the dominant part that the sense of hearing plays in one's Inner Life. In the inner life, the senses are reversed. Inner sight is a lower speed of vibration than inner sound. Mastering physical hearing and Shabda, Inner Hearing, is the key to Pratyahara. (Giri, 1976, p.212)

Swamiji also shares that "some of these Kriyas lead directly into deep concentration, and even meditative experiences can evolve out of the Pratyahara control" (Giri, 1976, p.212). Particularly at the beginning of one's Sadhana, however, the goal is to learn how to listen intently and without distractions and "not to grasp," not even at the hope of meditation.

Here are Swamiji's teachings in their integral form:

> 1. SHABDA KRIYA: Sit in any of the recommended Asana[23] and draw the thinking process into the Brow Center, Bhrumadhya Bindu. Listen for the loudest sound in the vicinity. Listen so intently to that sound that you become "one with it," so that the sound no longer exists as an independent entity. Then begin any form of Dharana concentration, or meditation of Dhyana. This listening to sound to achieve a Pratyahara may require listening to very quiet, even subtle sounds. Try choosing a sound which is not the loudest within your hearing, but "listen through" the loud sounds with intense concentration until the sound and you become one. Deep concentration can be achieved in this manner, much like a radio operator learning to listen to a signal through signals of other stations, atmospheric static and the usual environmental sounds.
>
> 2. SHABDA PRATYAHARA: Sit in any of the recommended postures and listen inside of your own head for the subtle sound of the blood coursing through the arteries and veins, the sound of blood pressure or the "flub-dub" of the heart's pulsation. Other body sounds may be used as well. Listen intently for two or three minutes, then allow the thinking/hearing to go outside of the body and listen for sounds right around the head. After listening

23 Among the recommended Asana for listening practices are Vajra Asana, Sukha Asana, Padma Asana. The details of these practices can be found in Chapter 4.

> for a few minutes, let the ears under the control of the mind listen in your immediate environment to sounds in the room or in the building or in the place where you sit. Now let the hearing go out into the area immediately around the site or building where you sit. Listen to every sound as it occurs. Now reach out with your hearing a hundred meters or so, perhaps up to a city block. Listen to any sounds occurring in that periphery. Stretch out the hearing for a mile, listening to all of the sounds circumscribed by the limits of your Pratyahara Kriya. Now let the thinking/hearing go as far away from you as humanly possible. Concentrate on sending the hearing to far-off distances: listen intently. In this way you have allowed the sense of hearing to do exactly what it has been created to do… to hear. Now having exercised the hearing to its fullest, withdraw the sense of hearing through a reversal of the steps of the Kriya, performing the true purpose of the Pratyahara at each stage until after ten to fifteen minutes, you re-enter the body again. Then listen intently to the subtle sounds within. Raise the mind with the last vestige of this inner concentration on sound into Bhrumadhya or Tisra Til or the Shiva Netra. These centres are included within the concept of Ajna Chakra, the Centre of Inspiration in Tantra, and Kundalini Yoga. (Giri, 1976, pp.211–212)

In the next chapter we will learn how the sound of the Guru of Gurus, Ishwara the Supreme Being, is AUM, the Mantra of Mantra, the Pranava Om, the vibration that existed before creation from which all other Mantras emerge.

Chapter 2

THE PRANAVA AUM

AUM is All that Is

The Sanskrit Mantra ॐ, transliterated in European languages as AUM, Aum, OṀ, or Oṁ, is the essential energy of the cosmos, a vibratory essence that existed before creation, and it is thus called Pranava (praṇava), from Nava ("new") and Pra-, "that which precedes anything else." Other names for this vibration are Omkara (oṁkara, "the sound of OṀ") and Udgeeta (udgītha, "the song from above"). Yogamaharishi Dr. Swami Gitananda Giri Guru Maharaj, in Lesson Seven of *Yoga: Step-by-Step*, shares how the AUM is at the root of the "Evolution of All Sounds":

> for to coin a name for God would require using the entire alphabet of every language belonging to every race, in every clime, in all times, past, now and still to come, plus the use of all ciphers, codes, gestures and meaningful symbols, yet, this could not be the name of God, for God must be more than any of this. God must be beyond the print of this page and the mind which conceives any idea of God in word, thought and symbol. At the end of futility, a single Pratika, a symbol, still remained, the last vestige of human reasoning. This Pratika stood as a sign post, pointing the way still higher upwards, hence, the term Pranava, "That which exists before ideation, mentation, mentalization, creation or birth of any form." Beyond the sign is the substance, the source, the goal: no words, no acts—stillness—inaudible, ineffable, AUM as experience. (Giri, 1976, p.28)

The identification of the Pranava with the Divine, Brahman, or Ishwara is present in the *Upanishads*[1] and other classical compositions of Yoga such as the *Bhagavad Gita*, the *Yoga Sutra*, and the *Shiva Purana* (śiva purāṇa). Para-Brahman is:

> the mighty energy of the universe that creates, and sustains, as well as evolves through change. This metaphysical principle of the universe is of the nature of pure existence, pure consciousness and pure bliss (sat cit ānandam). It is formless and not bound by the laws of space, time or causation. It is Nirguna, i.e. beyond the qualities of the three Gunas. (Bhavanani, 2005, p.17)

AUM is the goal, the instrument, and the process of returning into resonance with the essence of this pure consciousness.

Om in the Katha Upanishad

The *Katha Upanishad* (kaṭhopaniṣad) is found in the *Krishna Yajur Veda* (kṛṣṇa yajur veda) and teaches self-knowledge through the story of a young Brahmin, Nachiketa (nāciketa), and the presiding deity of death, Yama. Nachiketa wants to know about the Self[2] and asks Yama to teach him. Yama tries to dissuade him by offering worldly wealth and riches but the young Brahman does not waver. Finally, in Part 1, Chapter 2, Verses 15–17, after testing Nachiketa and finding him worthy of receiving such wisdom, Lord Yama teaches him about the OṀ, whose nature is beyond the past, the present, and the future, beyond thought and speech:

> [I:2:15]
>
> सर्वे वेदा यत्पदमामनन्ति
> तपांसि सर्वाणि च यद्वदन्ति ।
> यदिच्छन्तो ब्रह्मचर्यं चरन्ति
> तत्ते पदं संग्रहेण ब्रवीम्योमित्येतत् ॥ १५॥

---

1 The *Upanishads* are the concluding teachings of each *Veda*. The meaning of their name is "sitting by the feet of the teacher" and it comes from the modality through which they were received, orally from the mouth of the Rishi to the ear of the disciple (upa means "near," ni means "below" and refers to the feet of the Guru, and shat means "sitting"). There were thousands in origin and, while we have more than 200 written *Upanishads*, 108 of them are most revered.

2 The Self with a capital "s" is Brahman, or the absolute reality. The self with a lower "s" is each person's individual being.

sarve vedā yatpadamāmananti
tapāṁsi sarvāṇi ca yadvadanti
yadicchanto brahmacaryaṃ caranti
tatte padaṃ saṃgraheṇa bravīmyomityetat

[Yama said:] That goal which the Upanishads [the Veda] praise as the highest, which only austerities reveal, and which is won by those prepared to practice continence, I will briefly tell you what it is–it is Aum (Lokeswarananda, 1993, p.72).

[I:2:16]

एतद्ध्येवाक्षरं ब्रह्म एतद्ध्येवाक्षरं परम् ।
एतद्ध्येवाक्षरं ज्ञात्वा यो यदिच्छति तस्य तत् ॥ १६॥

etaddhyevākṣaraṃ brahma etaddhyevākṣaraṃ param
etaddhyevākṣaraṃ jñātvā yo yadicchati tasya tat

[Praising Aum and its worship, Yama said:] This akṣaram [Aum] is Brahman with attributes. This akṣaram [Aum] is also Brahman without attributes. He who knows this Aum can get whatever he wishes (Lokeswarananda, 1993, p.73).

[I:2:17]

एतदालम्बनँ श्रेष्ठमेतदालम्बनं परम् ।
एतदालम्बनं ज्ञात्वा ब्रह्मलोके महीयते ॥ १७॥

etadālambana~ śreṣṭhametadālambanaṃ param
etadālambanaṃ jñātvā brahmaloke mahīyate

Aum is the best way to attain Brahman. It is the way to attain both Brahman with attributes [Aparā Brahman] and Brahman without attributes [Parā Brahman]. The first leads you to Brahmaloka, where you enjoy the same status as Brahmā. The second leads you to union with Brahman (Lokeswarananda, 1993, p.74).

Om in the Bhagavad Gita

The *Bhagavad Gita*, the "Song Celestial," is a section of the classic Sanskrit epic, the *Mahabharata* (mahābhārata). While scholars still do not agree on this masterpiece's time of composition, with estimates varying from 1500 BCE to 200 CE, its teachings are considered immemorial and immortal and are attributed to the great sage Vyasa (vyāsaḥ). The oral traditions of India hold it to be at least 5000 years old, as the start of Kali Yuga is tied to the mortal transition of Lord Sri Krishna (kṛṣṇaḥ). The *Bhagavad Gita* consists of dialogues, arranged in 18 chapters (Adhyaya, adhyāya, lectures), for a total of 700 verses (śloka), between Lord Krishna and his disciple, the warrior Arjuna, on the battlefield of Kurukshetra (kurukṣetra). Krishna, an embodied avatar of Lord Vishnu (viṣṇu), is both the Godhead and Arjuna's charioteer. While the teachings are transmitted through the context of a story, they belong to humanity and have been revered by people of all spiritual traditions and parts of the world. Several are the teachings on the Pranava AUM. In Lecture 7, "Knowledge of the Absolute," we learn:

[7.8]

रसोऽहमप्सु कौन्तेय प्रभास्मि शशिसूर्ययो: |
प्रणव: सर्ववेदेषु शब्द: खे पौरुषं नृषु ||

raso 'ham apsu kaunteya prabhāsmi śhaśhi-sūryayoḥ
praṇavaḥ sarva-vedeṣhu śhabdaḥ khe pauruṣhaṁ nṛiṣhu

O son of Kunti, I am the taste of water, the light of the sun and the moon, the syllable om in the Vedic mantras; I am the sound in ether, and the ability in man (Prabhupāda, 1986, p.398).

Lecture 8, "Attaining the Supreme," details the importance of withdrawing our attention from the sense objects, "closing all the gates of the body," focusing the mind in the heart region, and drawing the life energy of Prana to the head through the process of Samyama:

[8.12]

सर्वद्वाराणि संयम्य मनो हृदि निरुध्य च |
मूर्ध्न्याधायात्मन: प्राणमास्थितो योगधारणाम् ||

sarva-dvārāṇi sanyamya mano hṛidi nirudhya cha
mūrdhnyādhāyātmanaḥ prāṇam āsthito yoga-dhāraṇām

The Yogic situation is that of detachment from all sensual engagements. Closing all the doors of the senses and fixing the mind on the heart and the life air at the top of the head, one establishes himself in yoga (Prabhupāda, 1986, p.454).

This state of "Yoga Dharana" is a prerequisite to "tune" into the inner Nada described in the following verse:

[8.13]

ओमित्येकाक्षरं ब्रह्म व्याहरन्मामनुस्मरन् |
यः प्रयाति त्यजन्देहं स याति परमां गतिम् ||

oṁ ityekākṣharaṁ brahma vyāharan mām anusmaran
yaḥ prayāti tyajan dehaṁ sa yāti paramāṁ gatim

After being situated in this yoga practice and vibrating the sacred syllable oṁ, the supreme combination of letters, if one thinks of the Supreme Personality of Godhead and quits his body, he will certainly reach the spiritual planets (Prabhupāda, 1986, p.455).

In Lecture 10, "The Opulence of the Absolute," we learn:

[10.25]

महर्षीणां भृगुरहं गिरामस्म्येकमक्षरम् |
यज्ञानां जपयज्ञोऽस्मि स्थावराणां हिमालयः ||

maharṣhīṇāṁ bhṛigur ahaṁ girām asmyekam akṣharam
yajñānāṁ japa-yajño 'smi sthāvarāṇāṁ himālayaḥ

Of the great sages I am Bhṛigu; of vibrations I am the transcendental oṁ. Of sacrifices I am the chanting of the holy names [japa], and of immovable things I am the Himālayas (Prabhupāda, 1986, p.571).

And, lastly, in Lecture 17, "The Divisions of Faith," we learn:

[17.23]

ॐ तत्सदिति निर्देशो ब्रह्मणस्त्रिविधः स्मृतः |
ब्राह्मणास्तेन वेदाश्च यज्ञाश्च विहिताः पुरा ||

oṁ tat sad iti nirdeśho brahmaṇas tri-vidhaḥ smṛitaḥ
brāhmaṇās tena vedāśh cha yajñāśh cha vihitāḥ purā

From the beginning of creation, the three words oṁ tat sat were used to indicate the Supreme Absolute Truth. These three symbolic representations were used by brahmaṇas while chanting the hymns of the Vedas and during sacrifices for the satisfaction of the Supreme (Prabhupāda, 1986, p.839).

[17.24]

तस्माद् ॐ इत्युदाहृत्य यज्ञदानतप:क्रिया: |
प्रवर्तन्ते विधानोक्ता: सततं ब्रह्मवादिनाम् ||

tasmād oṁ ity udāhṛitya yajña-dāna-tapaḥ-kriyāḥ
pravartante vidhānoktāḥ satataṁ brahma-vādinām

Therefore, transcendentalists undertaking performances of sacrifice, charity and penance in accordance with scriptural regulations begin always with oṁ, to attain the supreme (Prabhupāda, 1986, p.841).

Om in the Yoga Sutra

Maharishi Patanjali, in the 196 aphorisms of the *Yoga Sutra,* exposes human afflictions and their causes, the ways to overcome them until steadiness of body and mind are reached, and then the further steps to attain concentration (dhāraṇa), meditation (dhyāna), and finally, liberation (samādhi). The eight limbs (aṣṭāṅga) of Ashtanga Yoga are analyzed under many angles (aṅga) so that we may find our individual way into these codified disciplines. In Samadhi Pada (samādhi pāda), the first of the four parts (pāda), *Sutra* 27–29, Patanjali describes the benefit of the constant repetition of the Pranava Aum, the embodied vibratory form of the Absolute.

[I:27]

तस्य वाचकः प्रणवः ॥२७॥

tasya vācakaḥ praṇavaḥ

Pranava is the vibration of the Divine (Bhavanani, 2011a, p.71).

What this means is not that "the name of God is OṀ" but, rather, that OṀ is the closest human approximation to the causal vibration: "The Pranava is the name (vācakaḥ) of that divine state of existence that is omnipotent, omniscient and omnipresent" (Bhavanani, 2011a, p.71). When we evoke that vibration, we set up the ripple effect that travels from the gross, to the subtle, to the causal layer of existence. We cannot contemplate such a refined causal sound, as it is beyond our sensorial understanding, but we can create Its sound (śabda) through our vocal apparatus. When we evoke the Pranava (nāma), we tune in to the vibratory essence (rūpa) of Ishwara, a vibration beyond Karma (karma), our ego-based "doings," and Kleshas (kleśa), the challenges we encounter on our spiritual path:

[I:24]

क्लेशकर्मविपाकाशयैरपरामृष्टः पुरुषविशेष ईश्वरः ॥२४॥

kleśa karma vipāka-āśayaiḥ-aparāmṛṣṭaḥ puruṣa-viśeṣa īśvaraḥ

Ishwara is the special one beyond afflictions and the fructification of karma (Bhavanani, 2011a, p.68).

In the second part of the *Yoga Sutra*, Sadhana Pada (sādhana pāda), third aphorism, we learn about the Kleshas:

[II:3]

अविद्यास्मितारागद्वेषाभिनिवेशाः क्लेशाः ॥३॥

avidyā-asmitā-rāga-dveṣa-abhiniveśaḥ kleśāḥ

These afflictions are ignorance, false identity, attraction, repulsion and survival instinct (Bhavanani, 2011a, p.112).

The Kleshas surface when we are attached to life because of the fear of death. This sounds like a paradox at first, but it is a truth that we must contemplate. Our attractions, desires, repulsions, sense of "me and mine," and how we attach importance to name, fame, and status, at their root, surge from our need to survive. Fear of death inhibits our capacity to live life fully. Our understanding of life depends greatly on the concepts of space and time. Through cultural agreements on time, for example, we organize memories and create plans and projections. Through cultural agreements on space, we sustain constructs such as nationality and longing. When intoning the Mantra OṀ, we overcome the effects of these "obstacles of our practice." The repetition is not a mechanical one:

[I:28]

तज्जपस्तदर्थभावनम् ॥२८॥

taj-japas-tad-artha-bhāvanam

It must be chanted repeatedly with understanding and feeling (Bhavanani, 2011a, p.72).

One needs to first understand the meaning behind this seemingly simple one-syllable sound and then push one's mind beyond all understanding to vibrate with a devotional sentiment (bhāva) based on experience rather than creed. When chanted in this way, the Pranava becomes a tool to overcome the nine hindrances to Sadhana, the Antaraya (antarāyāḥ):

[I:29]

ततः प्रत्यक्चेतनाधिगमोऽप्यन्तरायाभावश्च ॥ २९ ॥

tataḥ pratyakcetanādhigamo'pyantarāyābhavaśca

This enables us to realize our true nature and removes the obstacles on the path (Bhavanani, 2011a, p.73).

[I:30]

व्याधि स्त्यान संशय प्रमादालस्याविरति भ्रान्तिदर्शनालब्ध
भूमिकत्वानवस्थितत्वानि चित्तविक्षेपास्तेऽन्तरायाः ॥ ३० ॥

vyādhi styāna saṁśaya pramādālasyāvirati bhrāntidarśanālabdha
bhūmikatvānavasthitatvāni cittavikṣepāte' antarāyāḥ

Illness, mental laziness, doubt, procrastination, sloth, sensual craving, false perception, inability to attain and maintain higher states are the mental obstacles (Bhavanani, 2011a, p.74)

The primitive consciousness from which these obstacles emerge is very strong. The chaotic vibration of their Vrittis creates dis-ease in our lives. The potent vibration of the OM, when repeated with discipline and abandon, "entrains" noise and results in a calming silence. The quietude of the mind is a prerequisite for spiritual life. The Rishis, Yogis, and spiritual masters have always praised the benefits of inner and outer silence as a form of self-control and regulation of impulses. Mauna, conscious inner and outer silence, is an observance and a restraint at the same time. By practicing silence, we learn to control our animalistic impulse to communicate at all times and learn to listen, especially to inner sound, by quieting the train of thoughts that are sometimes louder than our voice.

How Do We Evoke and Invoke the Pranava AUM?

We hope that the previous overview of some of the most important teachings of Sanatana Dharma may help contextualize the meaning of the Pranava Aum. The teachings of the Pranava are both culturally specific and intercultural. In Swamiji's words (Giri, 1976, p.20):

> Muslims use the AUM as OM-In (Amin) to invoke Allah and as a close to their prayers. The Christians use AUMEN (Amen) similarly. The Hebrew word for peacefulness, shalom (םולשׁ) is related to the concepts of perfection tied intrinsically to attributes of the Divine. In all religions a sign from God is called an OM-EN (Omen). To leave God out of your life is to OM-it (Omit) Him. As a supreme God, He is OM nilpotent (Omnipotent); He is OM-niscient, all-light, resplendent, effulgent, all knowing; He is OM-competent (Omcompetent), all-law; OM-nific (Omnific), all-creating; OM-nifarious (Omnifarious) in all things; Om-nigenous (Omnigenous) all kinds and species; He is OM-nipresent (Omnipresent), far as well as near, ubiquitous, being constantly met with; OM-nivorous (Omnivorous), He feeds on anything, even on Himself; OM-phalic (Omphalic), He is the Centre, the Hub of the Universe; He is the Lingam in the Yoni.

The teachings of Swami Gitananda on the Pranava AUM make this vast ocean of wisdom accessible to us in a step-by-step manner by rooting the metaphysical in the physical through the principles and practices of the Vibhaga Pranayama, sectional breathing, and the Pranava Pranayama. These are jewels of this Parampara and will reveal their luminescent strength and grace to those who practice them with devotion and respect.

The following quote from Swami Gitananda well expresses how valuable these teachings are:

> I feel in Kali Yuga, that the proper intonation and understanding of the Pranava AUM, the Mantra of Mantras, is actually enough for the modern Yoga Sadhak. The correct pronunciation can be taught to even those unskilled in languages. Many have described me as a teacher who bases his teachings on the Pranava, or on the sacred sound of AUM and to some extent, this is true. I teach a system of Pranava Pranayama, which was gifted to me by my Guru, as one of our basic spiritual practices. In this we link the basic sounds of "AAA," "OOO" and "MMM" to the breath moving in the various lobes of the lungs and the Hasta Mudras of Chin Mudra, Chinmaya Mudra,

> Adhi Mudra and Maha Mudra to help move Prana into the appropriate Nadis and air into the appropriate lung areas. I often remark that if my students did nothing but this Pranava Pranayama, with dedication and intensity with complete and pure one-pointedness of mind, they could achieve enlightenment. But of course, few take me seriously and most, despite my warnings, use it only as a "throw away" technique to open class sessions and personal Sadhana. (Giri, n.d., p.1)

Let's dive into the structural analysis of the Pranava to glimpse the enlightening correspondences between breathing and sonic articulation.

The syllable OṀ[3] is divided into three expressed sounds:

- the Akara Nada (akāra nāda)—the AAA sound representing creation
- the Ukara Nada (ūkāra nāda)—the UUU sound representing sustenance
- the Makara Nada (makāra nāda)—the MMM sound representing dissolution.

There is a fourth sound in the AUM: silence. This is not the silence described by "lack of sound." On the contrary, this is a peak of the practice of Nada Yoga, a silence that corresponds to the fourth level of consciousness, Turya (turya), Oneness with All that Is, or Samadhi. This resonance is not heard through the ears but in the center of the heart. It is the Anahata Nada.

The number three is sacred in many esoteric traditions. It is the number linked to creation and the manifestation of form. Yogacharya Dr. Ananda Balayogi Bhavanani in his book *Yoga 1 to 10* writes:

> The Pranava AUM (OM) is the Cosmic Nada (sacred sound of the universe), It existed before (Pra) anything arose anew (Nava). ... The Pranava consists of three parts, namely the Akara (AAA), the Ukara (UUU), and Makara (MMM). According to Tirumoolar,[4] the Akara stands for the Jiva, Ukara for the Para, and Makara for Shiva. He equates the Shivaya Mantra with the Pranava when he says that "Si" stands for Shiva, "Va" for Para, and "Ya" for

3 Due to the process of metaphony (guṇa sandhi), the change of a vowel sound brought about by assimilation to a preceding or following vowel, "A+U" in Sanskrit becomes "O."

4 Tirumoolar (Tirumular) was a Tamil Shaivite Yogi whose teachings form the *Tirumantiram* (also spelled *Tirumanthiram*), a sacred scripture of over 3000 verses whose name may be approximately translated as "Holy Incantation."

> the Jiva. According to the Yogatattvopanishad, the three Lokas, the three Vedas, the three Sandhyas, the three Svaras, the three Agnis, and the three Gunas are all supposed to be the letters of the Pranava. The Garuda Purana says that the three syllables represent the manifest (Vyakta), the unmanifest (Avayakta), and the Purusha. (Bhavanani, 2005, p.52)

When we repeat the Mantra in an audible way (japa), we manifest it at the level of Vaikhari, an expressed sound. When we intone the Mantra by contemplating it (ajapa), we manifest it at the level of Manasika (mānasika), very deep within the mind. In between, there is the Upanshu Japa (upāṃśu), a whispered repetition that is not audible to others externally but is audible to us. As an audible manifestation, the Pranava AUM involves a complete articulation of vowels and consonants as guttural, palatal, dental, labial, and cerebral. Here is what Swamiji writes about the metaphysical articulation of the AUM:

> AUM is the name of God in vibration, in sound. To intone the Pranava AUM, the "Mantra of Mantras," the "Sound of Sounds," is to intone, to evoke, the most potent of all powers in a Mantra, a vibratory rune. ... It is made up of three vibratory sounds- "A," "U," "M." The "A" (ah) is a guttural sound which must begin in the Manipura Chakra, the Solar Plexus, and is the lowest sound that can be produced by the human. The Pranava continues evolutionarily upwards on the out-going breath so that the "U" (ooh) emanates from the back of the throat, then along the tongue as a palatal sound, then continues forward against the teeth as a dental sound, and finally, as a labial sound at the lips. The final "M" (mmm) is sounded as the Pranava evolves upwards into the nose as a nasal vibration and finally reaches the height of sound evolution as a cerebral sound as it leaves the top of the skull. The sounding of the Pranava AUM thus encompasses every sound made by man. Therefore, it is thought to be a fitting term for God. The Pranava AUM is the most profound of Mantras, devoid of language inadequacy and semantically correct. (Giri, 1976, p.22)

The beginning sound of A, a guttural vowel, is condensed into the U and elevated in the last resonance of the M. Lastly, the tongue comes up in a cerebral retroflex sound which lifts the vibration to the top of the skull and beyond. The written letter that represents this sound is marked by the Chandra Bindu (candra bindu), a dot above a crescent ँ. This sound is elevated, physically, and it parallels our intention to elevate ourselves.[5] The upward movement of resonance corresponds to a rising of energy and subtlety of vibration, from the grossest to the subtler. Here is where the teachings of this Parampara share a gem: this upward movement contained in the correct articulation of the AUM corresponds to the natural breathing mechanics of our diaphragm and lungs. Our breathing is controlled by the autonomic nervous system and, luckily, we do not have to remember to inhale and exhale. This "gift" of evolution is also a tool to become aware of how we breathe. How do we breathe? Are we holding our breath when a trigger comes up? How do emotions alter our breathing patterns? The first step in Pranayama Sadhana and Mantra Yoga is to witness our breathing habits and to move from an instinctive and often erratic cycle of inhalation and exhalation to a human conscious control. In fact, it is from the sacred science of Mantra that certain Pranayama rhythms and counts emerged. When we change the way we breathe, we change the way we think; when we change the way we think, we change the way we perceive the world around us; when we change the way we perceive the world around us, the world around us begins to change in positive ways.

In any Mantra Japa, it is important to regulate the breath by counting the inhale and the exhale, Talam (tāla), the "rhythms," so that they become equal in length. Then we learn to prolong the breath, not by forcing but by relaxing. This is a breakthrough for many Yoga Sadhakas (yoga sādhaka) who hope to extend their breathing capacity by tensing the diaphragm, the intercostal muscles, abdominal muscles, and back muscles. While muscular activity is essential in Pranayama, no tension is required. One's breathing capacity is directly proportional to the level of homeostasis, the balance between the sympathetic (active) and parasympathetic (receptive) nervous system.[6] One needs to be aware, active, and completely relaxed to breathe in a Yogic way. Vice versa, slow, deep and conscious breathing may regulate our autonomic nervous system, activating the parasympathetic functions of the vagus nerve and resulting in a sense of ease and calm. Equipped with the twin qualities of Abhyasa (abhyāsa), steady practice, and Vairagya, dispassion towards failure

---

5 At Ananda Ashram, Sanskrit is taught, as part of Yoga Sadhana, by Yogacharini Devasena Bhavanani, the Dharmapatni (wife and spiritual companion) of Yogacharya Dr. Ananda Balayogi Bhavanani. By learning the articulation of Sanskrit phonemes, students learn how to invoke Mantras with the correct pronunciation and how to resonate the Pranava AUM in various parts of the vocal and nasal cavity.

6 This topic will be developed in Chapter 4.

or success, we may reach the fourth stage, the Kevala Kumbhaka (kevala kumbhaka), an automatic breath retention that signifies "the beginning of the higher controls that are called Prana Jnana Kriyas" (Giri, 2008, p.60).[7]

The quality of Om Japa, especially when uttered in expressed sound, follows the refinement of one's breathing awareness and capacity. Vocal sounds originate in the area of the navel (nābhi), connected in Tantra to Manipura Chakra (maṇipūra chakra) at the solar plexus. This area corresponds, in our physical body, to the diaphragmatic region. What is the spiritual meaning of the solar plexus? The solar plexus connects us to the center of the Universe through a psychic umbilical cord, just like a baby is connected to the mother by a physical umbilical cord. When we breathe in a conscious manner and intone a chant, the feel-good hormones such as endorphins, enkephalins, serotonin, and oxytocin are secreted. Our "gut" produces over 95 percent of serotonin and, according to scientific research:

> The gut-brain axis is a bidirectional communication network that links the enteric and central nervous systems. This network is not only anatomical, but it extends to include endocrine, humoral, metabolic, and immune routes of communication as well. The autonomic nervous system, hypothalamic-pituitary-adrenal (HPA) axis, and nerves within the gastrointestinal (GI) tract, all link the gut and the brain, allowing the brain to influence intestinal activities, including activity of functional immune effector cells; and the gut to influence mood, cognition, and mental health. (Appleton, 2018, p.28)

When we invoke the Pranava AUM, together with physical, emotional, and mental health, we positively influence our spiritual health. Spiritual health has been defined:

> as a state of being where an individual is able to deal with day-to-day life issues in a manner that leads to the realization of one's full potential, meaning and purpose of life and fulfillment from within. Such a state of being is attainable through self-evolution, self-actualisation and transcendence. Existing literature reveals that spirituality broadly focuses on being deeply involved in day-to-day activities of the world, at the same time being detached, where

7 On the previous page, Swamiji warns the practitioners that advanced Kumbhakas are dangerous for beginners and that "they should be perfected only under a Guru as they involve prolonged periods of breath retention" (Giri, 2008, p.59).

> there is a continuous effort for developing universality of love, compassion and equanimity to replace anger, jealousy, ego and hatred, resulting in utilization of one's abilities to the fullest and even transcending beyond that. It unfolds the process of "Becoming" to "Being" and extending "Beyond" to attain fullest positive health. (Dhar *et al.*, 2013, p.3)

This is what the *Upanishads* and other ancient teachings have been inspiring us to understand and practice all along. "Yoga is a way of life" taught Swamiji, and our life, without breathing, is not sustainable.

Vibhaga Pranayama: Micro-Lobular Breathing

The respiratory diaphragm is a huge dome-shaped muscle that divides our thoraco-abdominal cavity into two halves, the thoracic (chest) cavity and the abdominal cavity. The main nerves that control the movement of the diaphragm are the two phrenic nerves, which originate from the cervical area of C3–5. The diaphragm attaches at the costal muscles along the lower ribcage, high in the front at the sternum, and deep in the back along the spine, and it also attaches to itself by a central tendon which allows a safe passage for the aorta, the vena cava, and the esophagus.

Our inhalation occurs thanks, mainly, to the contraction of the diaphragm and its downward and upward excursions in the thoracic-abdominal cavity. It is not our inhale that lowers the diaphragm; rather, it is the "lowering" of this muscle through its contraction and downward excursion that creates an increase in anterior-posterior, vertical, and transverse dimensions of the thoracic cavity, creating a "space" for the "in-breath" to occur. When we inhale, the lung's pleura that is attached to the diaphragmatic pleura lowers too, in turn activating the intercostal muscles to contract and increase the stretch out. At the same time, we consciously activate the accessory muscles to pull up—all of this results in an increased intrathoracic volume. With this increase in volume, the intrathoracic pressure inside the chest decreases and air is automatically sucked into the thorax through the nose and/or mouth. The whole process is driven by intrinsically manipulated pressure-volume changes. It thus may be surprising to learn that we do not really breathe "from" the mouth or nose. We breathe through them thanks to the pressure-volume changes in the chest cavity resulting from contraction and relaxation of the diaphragm.

Our respiratory system consists of two lungs, with the right lung having three lobes and the left having two. Each of these lobes has smaller subdivisions of two to five bronchopulmonary segments. There are ten such segments in each lung: the upper lobes have three, the middle lobe (on the right) and lingula (on the left) have two, while the lower lobes on both sides have five. On both sides the upper lobes have segments named apical, posterior, and anterior, while the lower lobes have the superior (apical) and four basal segments (anterior, medial, posterior, and lateral). Each of the ten has an independent arterial and venous supply, nervous supply, lymphatic supply, and air supply.

From the Yogic perspective, it is considered that we have three subsections (vibhāga) in each of the three areas (low, mid, and upper) of the lungs. This makes a total of nine areas (front low, side low, back low; front mid, side mid, back mid; front upper, side upper, back upper), which is uncannily similar to the ten bronchopulmonary segmental concept of modern medical science. Vibhaga Pranayama is an exploration of each section and its subsections of front, side, and back, resulting in nine-part sectional breathing. Swami Gitananda, in *Yoga: Step-by-Step*, Lesson Three, wrote that "Vibhaga Pranayama, Sectional or Lobular Breathing, is the 'A, B, C' of Pranayama and is the beginning of good breath control. Without positive, physical control of the three major sections of each lung, real control will not exist" (Giri, 1976, p.11). The lungs are divided into three major sections:

- Adham, the inferior or lower chest, abdominal area
- Madhyam, the mid, thoracic, or intercostal area
- Adhyam, the superior, high, or clavicular area.

To become more aware of these sections, and focus our minds, we use the Sparsha Mudra (sparśa mudrā), a "sealing touch," to activate a gentle reflexogenic impulse between the palm and fingers of the hands and each of the sections, i.e. lower (front, side, and back), middle (front, side, and back), and upper (front, side, and back). The hands are an extension of the heart and the Heart Center, Anahata Chakra. The fingers should be gently kept together so that the hands are touching only one subsection of the lungs.

Touching different parts of the chest reminds us that we have various sections of the lungs in which to breathe. As the ancient saying goes, "yato mana, tathā prāṇa," "Where the mind goes, Prana flows." The reflexogenic effect of the Mudra has effects on our nervous system, benefitting all of our other systems. The area in the brain that is dedicated to the hands, the insula, is big, and its functions are linked to the experience of desires, cravings, and addictions. Its dysfunctions are related to neuropsychiatric disorders. When we use the Sparsha Mudra, we are experiencing a focusing of the flow of Prana into specific bronchopulmonary segments, resulting in a self-directed neuroplasticity that creates pathways to change our self-awareness.

1 - Front, 2 - Side, 3 - Back (not shown)

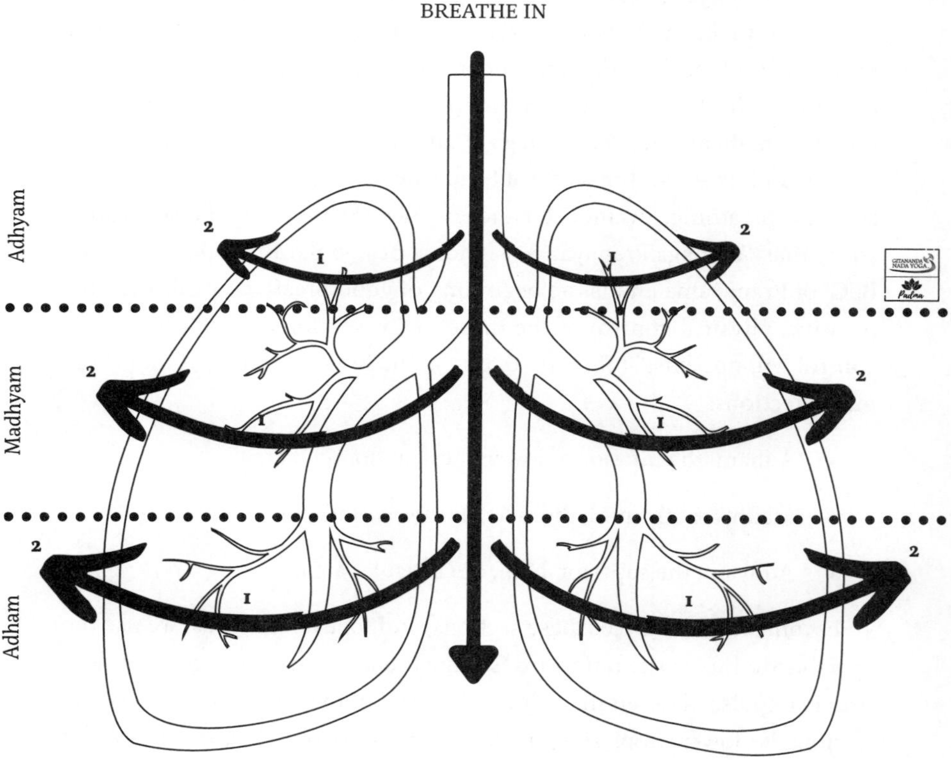

Vibhaga Pranayama Inhalation
A color version of this image can be downloaded from uk.singingdragon.com/catalogue/book/9781839974502.

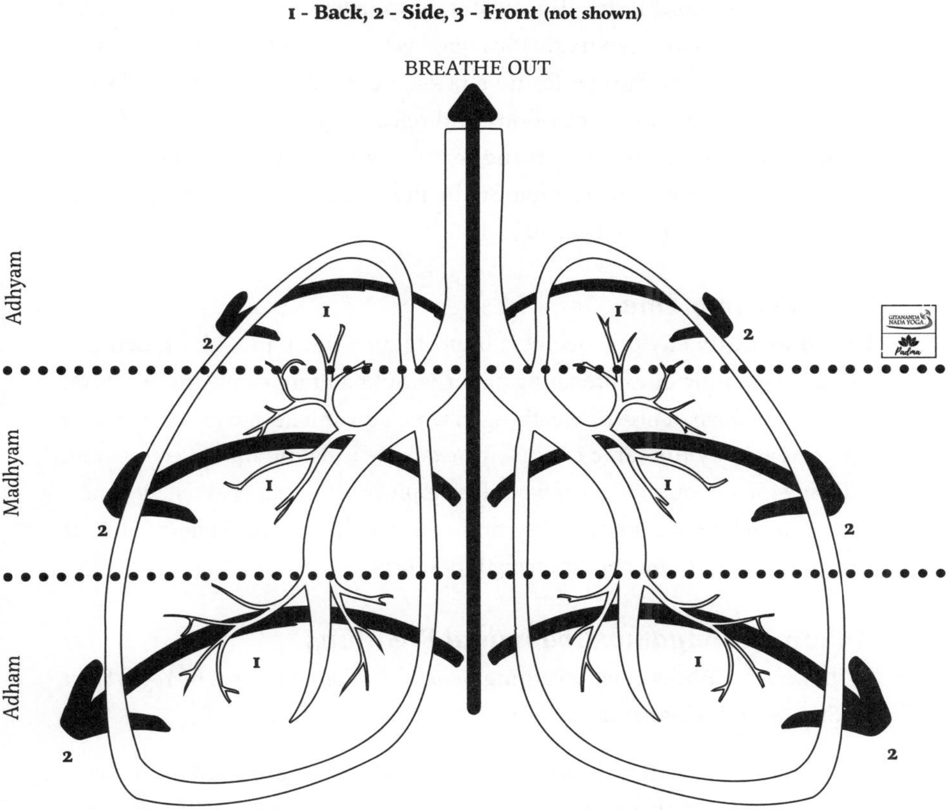

Vibhaga Pranayama Exhalation
A color version of this image can be downloaded from uk.singingdragon.com/catalogue/book/9781839974502.

How to Practice[8]

Vajra Asana

In Gitananda Yoga, Pranayama is performed from the posture of Vajra Asana, the "Adamantine Posture," which symbolizes, and contains, the energy of the

8 Authors' note: This is a general sketch of a basic technique taught in Rishiculture Ashtanga Yoga and is not intended as an instruction in this method of Pranava Breathing. Those interested in this practice would do well to contact a competent teacher trained in this method. This Pranava Pranayama is also taught in *Yoga: Step-by-Step*, the Yoga Correspondence Course authored by Yogamaharishi Dr. Swami Gitananda and, since 2020, available online through ICYER. Video tutorials are available on the YouTube channels of Dr. Ananda and Dr. Sangeeta (see the section "To Learn More…" for links).

thunderbolt of Lord Indra. This posture is excellent for grounding and for making sure that the diaphragmatic region is free from unnecessary pressure or constraints. If you can't perform Vajra Asana, any sitting position will work as long as you can align your body and release any unnecessary pressure from the area of the diaphragm and torso. Begin to calm your thoughts by regulating your breath in a simple Sukha Pranayama (inhaling on counts of six and exhaling on counts of six).

Sukha Pranayama

Before we begin any practice, it is important to check in with oneself and to start regulating one's breathing patterns. Sukha Pranayama, the "Pleasant Breath," is a form of nostril breathing in which the inhale and exhale patterns are regulated by the same counts, for example inhaling for six counts and exhaling for six counts. This apparently simple practice offers excellent results such as a feeling of calm, stability, and ease. Its physiological effects include slowing the heart rate and lowering blood pressure.

Adham Pranayama: Abdominal Breathing

In the section "Abdominal Breathing Benefits" of Lesson Three of *Yoga: Step-by-Step*, Swami Gitananda writes:

> Abdominal breathing is the natural form of breathing ordered by the automatic of vegetative part of your nervous system. Ladies are usually poor abdominal breathers and suffer as a consequence. Abdominal breathing governs the flow of Prana below the navel, so if this form of breathing is faulty, all sorts of negative conditions appear, such as: painful, irregular, heavy or scanty menstrual flow, hemorrhoids and varicose veins of the legs, oedema or water retention in the knees and ankles, phlebitis or inflammation of the lining of the veins, and cold feet through faulty circulation. In a man these conditions are also the result of faulty abdominal breathing. Men usually are good abdominal breathers. Adham Pranayama will correct these conditions.
>
> The Pranic flow in Abdominal Breathing, the Adham Pranayama, influences the blood circulation into the sacral and pelvic area and down into the legs. As the blood is propelled out from the mighty heart pump, it moves in three distinct and separate pathways: one, to the lower body and legs; two, to the heart muscles and the arms; three, to the neck and head. Buried

deep within the cells of the lungs are special reflexo-genic "feedback" nerves which are only stimulated by exaggerated deep inspirations and expirations. Normal breathing does not stimulate these receptors. When stimulated, these receptors send signals back to the respiratory center within the human brain, conditioning that center to perfect breathing. (Giri, 1976, p.12)

PRACTICE

Find your sternum, the bone at the center of your chest, and then, below it, the floating ribs. Place your hands gently together pointing towards the sternum on your floating ribs. Relax your shoulders down, roll your head, and shake your head to make sure you are not holding any unnecessary tension. Keep your fingers together, including your thumbs.

Adham: Front

1. Exhale to prepare.
2. Breathe in and out through the nose and feel the hands move as you inhale and exhale.
3. Inhale 1-2-3-4-5-6, exhale 1-2-3-4-5-6.
4. Inhale, imagine the diaphragm coming down, exhale 1-2-3-4-5-6.
5. Inhale… exhale…
6. Repeat for a total of nine rounds.
7. Relax and witness yourself.

Adham: Side

From the front, we move to the side of the lower section of the lungs, Adham Pranayama. Keep your shoulders relaxed as best as you can.

1. Exhale to prepare.
2. Breathe in and out through the nose and feel the hands move as you inhale and exhale.
3. Inhale 1-2-3-4-5-6, exhale 1-2-3-4-5-6.

4. Inhale… exhale… shoulders down, lips relaxed.
5. Inhale… exhale…
6. Repeat for a total of nine rounds.
7. Relax and witness yourself.

Adham: Back

Moving backwards, we're going to do a rotation of the hands so that you can feel the back of your lungs with the palm of the hands, which have a full reflexogenic capacity. Keep the fingers together, pointing towards the vertebral column. Relax the posture.

1. Exhale to prepare.
2. Breathe in and out through the nose and feel the hands move as you inhale and exhale.
3. Inhale 1-2-3-4-5-6, exhale 1-2-3-4-5-6.
4. Inhale… exhale…
5. Inhale… exhale…
6. Repeat for a total of nine rounds.
7. Relax and witness yourself.

Adham: Front, Side, and Back

Next, let's practice "front, side, and back" as one inhale, and "back, side, and front" as one exhale. We breathe in from the front and exhale from the back because of our physical anatomy. Like a pair of bellows, when we inhale, the intercostal muscles "open up," starting at the front. As we exhale, the diaphragm relaxes, the intercostal muscles contract, and we "close up." We will keep a 6x6 count: inhaling 1-2 front, 3-4 side, 5-6 back; exhaling from the back 1-2, side 3-4, front 5-6. Everything else is relaxed as best as we can.

1. Exhale to prepare.
2. Breathe in and out through the nose and feel the hands move as you inhale and exhale.

3. Inhale 1-2, side 3-4, back 5-6, exhale back 1-2, side 3-4, front 5-6.
4. Inhale… exhale from the back-side-front.
5. Repeat for a total of nine rounds.
6. Relax and witness yourself.

Madhyam Pranayama: Mid-Chest Breathing

In the section "Madhyam Pranayama: Intercostal Breathing Benefits" of Lesson Four of *Yoga: Step-by-Step*, Swami Gitananda writes:

> Mid-breathing or Intercostal breathing requires conscious mental control to perfect. It is not a normal part of the autonomic breathing function. Ladies are generally good mid-breathers because of the shape of their chest and the position of the breasts. Men are poor breathers in this area and require a great deal of training to be able to breathe easily around and behind the heart. Because of this, men suffer more from heart conditions than women. Ninety-five out of one hundred cases of heart disease affect men. Madhyam Pranayama governs the flow of air and Prana into the mid-chest and heart area, while the action of the breath diminishes the fat around the heart which accumulates through faulty breathing in this same area. A minimum of six minutes per day should be spent on this form of mid-breathing to open up the cells of the lungs normally not used. It is an excellent way to prevent heart disease and for those already affected, the only way in which the condition can be permanently alleviated. (Giri, 1976, pp.15–16)

PRACTICE

Let's move to the middle section of the lungs, Madhyam Pranayama. The principles and practice are the same, only we now focus on the three areas of the middle section of the lungs. Bring your hands to the pectoral area of your lungs. Shoulders down and back, elbows and arms slightly away from the torso to allow for expansion of the lungs.

Madhyam: Front

1. Exhale to prepare.
2. Breathe in and out through the nose and feel the hands move as you inhale and exhale.
3. Inhale 1-2-3-4-5-6, exhale 1-2-3-4-5-6.
4. Inhale… exhale…
5. Inhale… exhale…
6. Repeat for a total of nine rounds.
7. Relax and witness yourself.

Madhyam: Side

From the pectoral front, we move to the pectoral side; this is higher than earlier.

1. Exhale to prepare.
2. Breathe in and out through the nose and feel the hands move as you inhale and exhale.
3. Inhale 1-2-3-4-5-6, exhale 1-2-3-4-5-6.
4. Inhale… exhale…
5. Inhale… exhale…
6. Repeat for a total of nine rounds.
7. Relax and witness yourself.

Madhyam: Back

From the side we move to the back. This position may be a bit challenging. Simply do your best.

1. Exhale to prepare.
2. Breathe in and out through the nose and feel the hands move as you inhale and exhale.

3. Inhale 1-2-3-4-5-6, exhale 1-2-3-4-5-6.
4. Inhale… exhale…
5. Inhale… exhale…
6. Repeat for a total of nine rounds.
7. Relax and witness yourself.

Madhyam: Front, Side, and Back

Let's connect the three sections of Madhyam Pranayama together, the three minor sections of the mid section of the lungs, so the front, the side, and the back of Madhyam Pranayama.

1. Exhale to prepare.
2. Breathe in and out through the nose and feel the hands move as you inhale and exhale.
3. Inhale 1-2, side 3-4, back 5-6, exhale back 1-2, side 3-4, front 5-6.
4. Inhale… exhale from the back-side-front.
5. Repeat for a total of nine rounds.
6. Relax and witness yourself.

Adhyam Pranayama: Apical Breathing

In the section "Adhyam Pranayama: Clavicular Breathing" of Lesson Five of *Yoga: Step-by-Step*, Swami Gitananda teaches:

> The high or clavicular breath which fills the apical segments of the lungs requires conscious mental control as it is not a normal part of the autonomic breathing function. Very few people breathe properly in these high lobes, accounting for the tragic number of asthmatic and sinus type breathers. Adhyam Pranayama governs the flow of air and Prana into the high chest area. The Prana filling this area controls all sorts of breathing difficulties, as well as many allergies affecting the poor breather. Because of the lower position of the bronchial tubes supplying air to the upper lobes, these lobes often remain partially filled with stale, residual air that can only be emptied by continuous, conscious Adhyam Pranayama. Conscious effort should be

taken to do this Pranayama at least six minutes per day to open up the cells of the lungs not normally used. Those suffering from dyspnoea, or difficult breathing, will get relief almost immediately and with a conscious use of all three forms of the Vibhaga Pranayama, breathing difficulties will soon be a thing of the past. (Giri, 1976, p.A-17)

PRACTICE

Let's continue to the apical upper section of the lungs. Place your hand under the collarbones, fingers together. Here, find the collarbones and lift your hands, with the fingers together, and place them right under the collarbones. That's where the upper sections of the lungs are. We will breathe here in the same way as we have breathed for the previous areas.

Adhyam: Front

1. Exhale to prepare.
2. Breathe in and out through the nose and feel the hands move as you inhale and exhale.
3. Inhale… exhale…
4. Inhale… exhale…
5. Inhale… exhale…
6. Repeat for a total of nine rounds.
7. Relax and witness yourself.

Adhyam: Side

Next, become aware of the side of the upper lungs—right under your armpit. Place your hands on your thighs. Imagine you're like a beautiful container, a jar, and that this whole section is free to breathe. Shoulders are down and back.

1. Exhale to prepare.
2. Breathe in and out through the nose and feel the hands move as you inhale and exhale.

3. Inhale… exhale…
4. Inhale, relax your lips, relax your chin… exhale…
5. Inhale… exhale…
6. Repeat for a total of nine rounds.
7. Relax and witness yourself.

Adhyam: Back

Lift your arms over the head, bend your elbows, and place your hands on the upper back section of the lungs, right on the trapezius muscles. Keep your focus here. It may be possible that you won't feel much movement here at the beginning. This sensation will improve with a steady and relaxed practice.

1. Exhale to prepare.
2. Breathe in and out through the nose and feel the hands move as you inhale and exhale.
3. Inhale… exhale…
4. Inhale… exhale…
5. Inhale… exhale…
6. Repeat for a total of nine rounds.
7. Relax and witness yourself.

Adhyam: Front, Side, and Back

Let's connect the three subsections of the upper section of the lungs.

1. Exhale to prepare.
2. Breathe in and out through the nose and feel the hands move as you inhale and exhale.
3. Inhale 1-2, side 3-4, back 5-6, exhale back 1-2, side 3-4, front 5-6.
4. Inhale… exhale from the back-side-front.
5. Repeat for a total of nine rounds.

6. Relax and witness yourself.

Let's take a moment to trace back the journey we have made together from the Adham, Madhyam, Adhyam, in the nine parts front-side-back, front-side-back, front-side-back. Let the teaching and the practice sit with you for a moment before we continue.

Mahat Yoga Pranayama: Full Yogic Breathing

We are now ready to perform the "Grand Complete Yogic Breath" filling all three sections of the lungs in their totality. Let's read Swamiji's instructions from *Yoga: Step-by-Step*, Lesson Six:

> to aid in gaining positive control over these three breathing areas, place one hand onto the diaphragmatic region, the second hand at mid-chest. The lower hand may be raised to the high chest area after the lower lobes are filled, or one may concentrate with the mind into the high lobes. With the hands in the recommended position, start a long, deep breath regulating at least one third of the time of the breath to the abdominal area, then continuing the breath into the mid chest for another third of the time allotted, then finally filling the high clavicular area of the chest in the remaining one third of the count. For a beginner, a "two count" into each of the lung areas is recommended so that the breath comes two times two times two (2x2x2) until the Complete or Grand Yoga Breath is attained. The breath should be held in for a short period of time before being discharged in the same order and timing as the incoming breath (2x2x2). That is, the breath is let out from the lower lobes first, then the middle lobes, then, finally, the upper lobes. One should also see that the outgoing breath in each section is let out from the back lobes first, then the side lobes, and lastly from the front lobes. (Giri, 1976, p.23)

This breathing pattern forms a double helix which, symbolically, represents the spiraling movement of the Pingala Nadi (piṅgala nadī) and the Ida Nadi (iḍā nadī) around the Sushumna Nadi as seen in the illustrations below.

1 - Lower Front, 2 - Lower Side, 3 - Lower Back
4 - Middle Front, 5 - Middle Side, 6 - Middle Back
7 - Upper Front, 8 - Upper Side, 9 - Upper Back

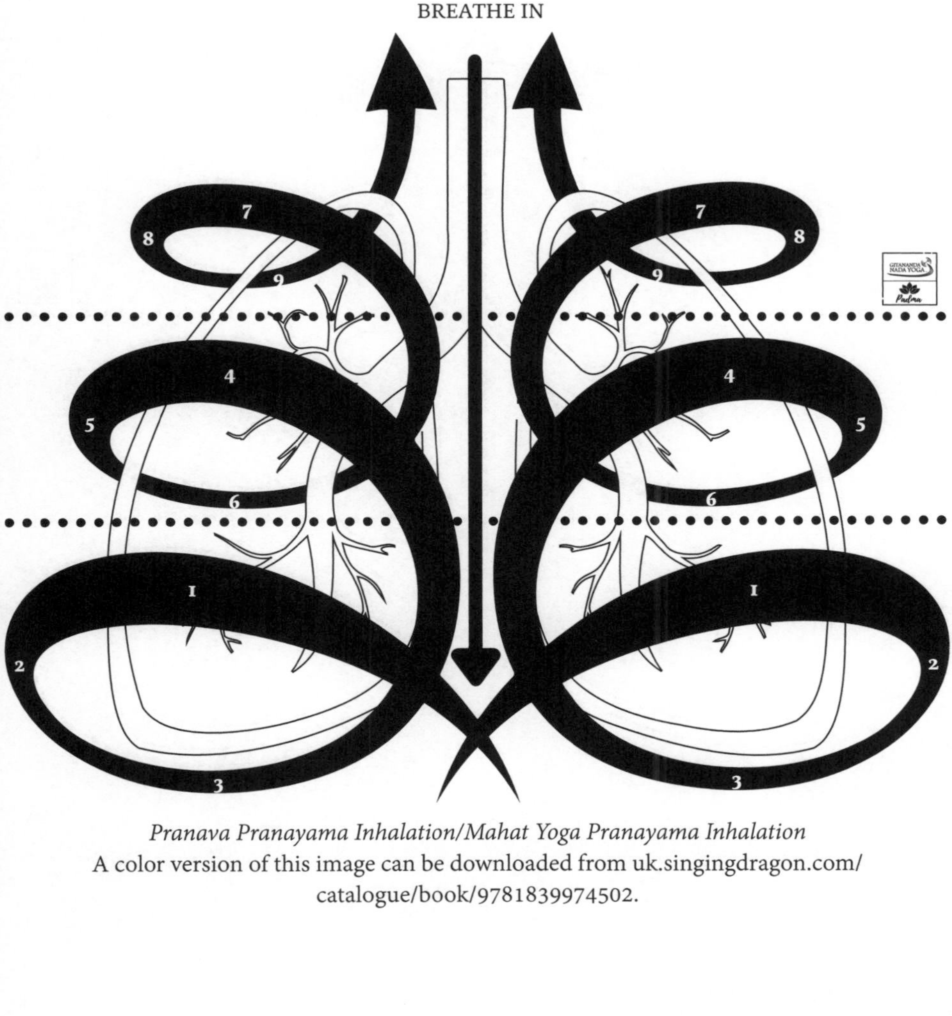

Pranava Pranayama Inhalation/Mahat Yoga Pranayama Inhalation
A color version of this image can be downloaded from uk.singingdragon.com/catalogue/book/9781839974502.

1 - Lower Back, 2 - Lower Side, 3 - Lower Front
4 - Middle Back, 5 - Middle Side, 6 - Middle Front
7 - Upper Back, 8 - Upper Side, 9 - Upper Front

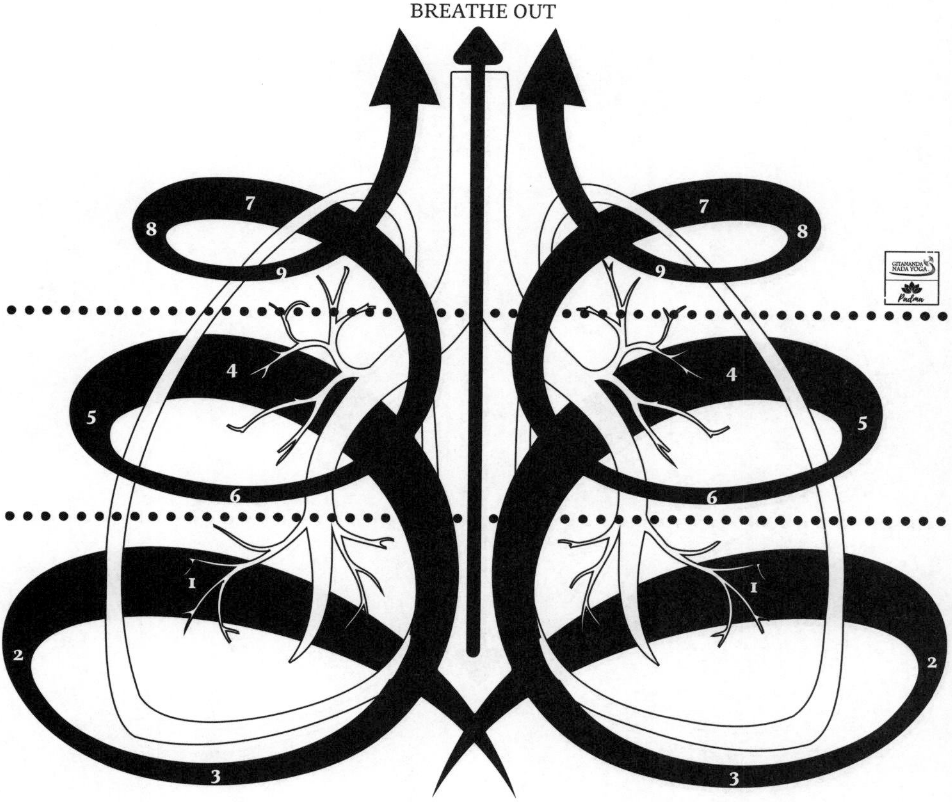

Pranava Pranayama Exhalation/Mahat Yoga Pranayama Exhalation
A color version of this image can be downloaded from uk.singingdragon.com/catalogue/book/9781839974502.

PRACTICE

Inhalation: the movement of the in-breath is a spiraling, upwards movement in a double helical spiral *from front to back*: Adham Pranayama, front-side-back; Madhyam Pranayama, front-side-back; Adhyam Pranayama, front-side-back).

Here, Swamiji recommends performing the Aprakasha Mudra, a "swallowing of the breath action" after the incoming breath to avoid a bronchospasm (Giri, 1976, p.23).

Exhalation: the movement of the out-breath is a spiraling, upwards movement in a double helical spiral *from back to front*: Adham Pranayama, back-side-front; Madhyam Pranayama, back-side-front; Adhyam Pranayama, back-side-front.

Vibhaga Pranayama with Hasta Mudras

After practicing for a while, and after developing awareness of the nine regions in each lung with the gentle touch of the Sparsha Mudra, we begin practicing with the Hasta Mudras, specific hand gestures that create an energy seal. Hasta Mudras are a subtle language expressing our intent to direct our energy in a certain way for a certain purpose. There is a Shloka in Bharatanatyam, the classical Southern Indian dance form, that teaches us:

यतो हस्त स्ततो दृष्टि यतो दृष्टि स्ततो मनः
यतो मनः स्ततो भाव: यतो भाव स्ततो रस:

yato hasta stato dṛṣṭi, yato dṛṣṭi stato manah
yato manah stato bhāva, stato bhāva stato rasa

Where your hands go your eyes go,
where your eyes go your mind goes,
where your mind goes the feeling evolves,
where the feeling evolves the rasa flows.

The Hasta Mudras of Vibhaga and Pranava Pranayama create reflexogenic messages that are sent to the brainstem, the respiratory center which, in yoga, is called Aprakasha Bindu (aprakāśa bindu). In the Aprakasha Bindu there are three subsidiary Bindus: Adhama Bindu at the bottom of the stem, Madhyama Bindu in the middle, and Adhyama Bindu at the top. Chin Mudra (cit mudrā) stimulates Adhama Bindu, Chinmaya Mudra (chinmaya mudrā) stimulates Madhyama Bindu, and Adhi Mudra (ādhi mudrā) stimulates Adhyam Bindu, resulting in a fuller and more complete respiration in the related sections of the lungs. The Hasta Mudras of Vibhaga and Pranava Pranayama are named in correspondence to the Bindu they stimulate: Chin Mudra for Adham Pranayama, the Chinmaya Mudra for Madhyam Pranayama, the Adhi Mudra for Adhyam Pranayama, and the Brahma Mudra (brahmā mudrā) for Mahat Yoga Pranayama.

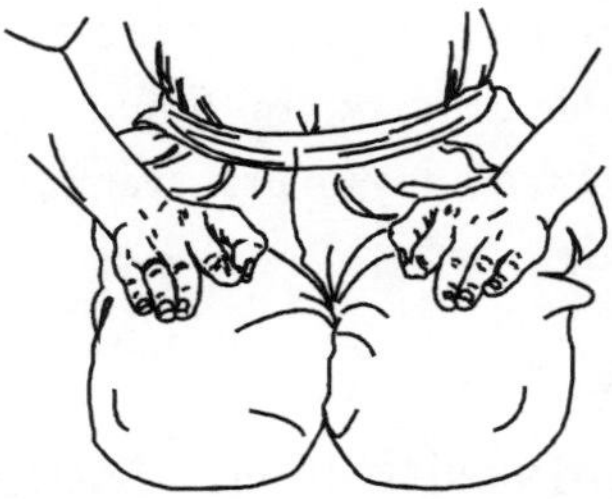

Chin Mudra

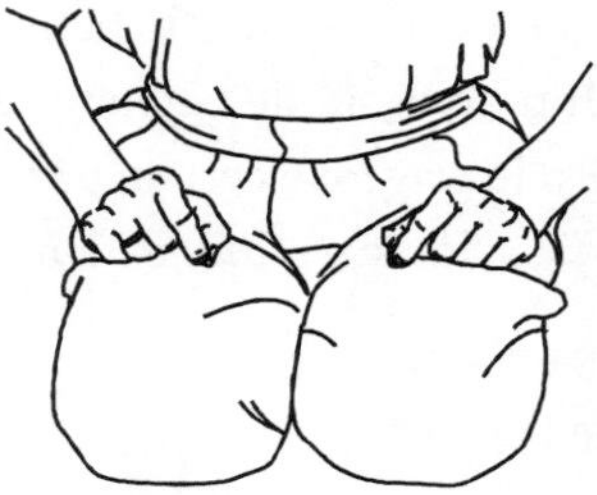

Chinmaya Mudra

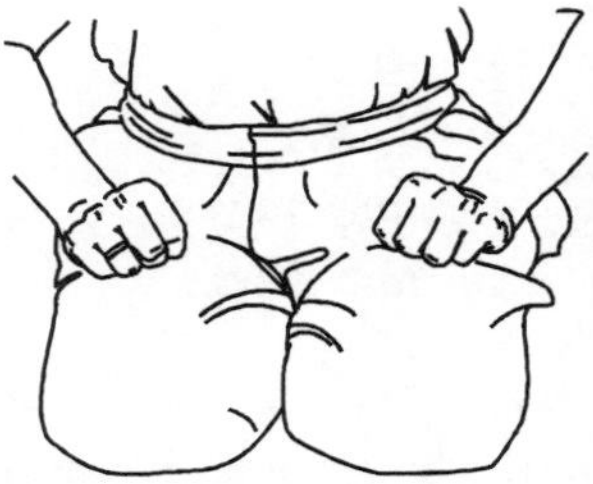

Adhi Mudra

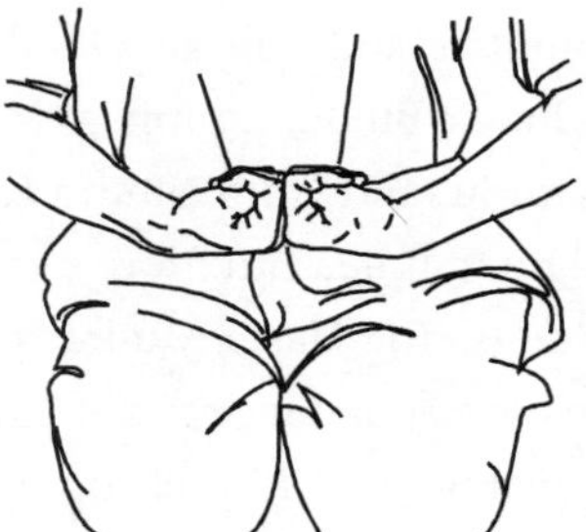

Brahma Mudra

Vibhaga and Pranava Pranayama Hasta Mudras

Mudras connect certain sections of the fingers with concepts: for example, the thumb is associated with Universality and the Divine; the index finger with Individuality and the self; the other three fingers with the Gunas, the essential qualities of nature, and the Doshas (doṣa), the bodily humors. Fingers also correspond to planets and other symbols. Ammaji Yogacharini Meenakshi Devi Bhavanani teaches us that Mudras are gestures of intrapersonal, interpersonal, and transpersonal communication. Intrapersonal refers to communication within the self; interpersonal refers to communication with an external environment, including other people, animals, objects, and ideas; transpersonal communication refers to communication with something greater than us, however we may name that intelligence force that sustains life.

Swami Gitananda codified this wisdom in a practical system of correspondences as follows:

- Intrapersonal Communication: Chin Mudra (Adham Pranayama, Abdominal Section of the Lungs), the Gesture of Consciousness (Chit = consciousness; "T" + "M" = N). In this Mudra, the tip of the thumb and index finger touch, creating a circle, while the other fingers are kept straight and relaxed. We make a mindful effort to unite individuality with universality, while keeping the other three fingers restrained, representing the three Gunas (guṇa) and the three Doshas, aspects of the gross, subtle, and causal layers of existence.

- Interpersonal Communication: Chinmaya Mudra (Madhyam Pranayama, Middle Section of the Lungs), Gesture of Binding the Self to Consciousness (cit + maya). In this Mudra, the tip of the thumb and index finger touch, creating a circle, while the other fingers are curled with the tips touching the center of the palms. We begin a process of Pratyahara, of controlling the stimuli of senses and bringing our awareness towards inner reality.

- Transpersonal Communication: Adhi Mudra (Adhyam Pranayama, Apical Section of the Lungs), the Gesture of Binding Oneself with the Divine. In this Mudra, the thumb is bent and brought towards the center of the palm, while the other fingers gently close around it, making a soft fist around the thumb. The thumb represents the Divine, and in this gesture we remember that the Divine is hidden by all the aspects of the senses and the illusionary world. Adhi Mudra is the Mudra of the highest (adhi) causal source.

Adham Pranayama with the Chin Mudra (Cit Mudrā, the Gesture of Consciousness)

When adding the Hastha Chin Mudra, gently press the thumb and index finger together and allow the other fingers to relax. Place the palms down on your inner thighs, close to the hips, to create a close circuit in the energy flow from the cervical brachial plexus and the lumbosacral plexus. With the mudra, we are sending reflexogenic feedback to the brainstem neurons of the Chin Bindu in the Aprakasha Bindu to focus on the lower area of the lungs. This is a message of intrapersonal communication. The dull and heavy nature of my mind (tamas) is balanced. This practice benefits the lower part of the body, below the abdominal region, and the gross body, the Sthula Sharira.

Madhyama Pranayama with Chinmaya Mudra (Maya Means "To Bind," Gesture of Binding Yourself into Consciousness)

When adding the Hastha Mudra, from the Chin Mudra, curl the fingers and create the Chinmaya Mudra, and place them on the inner thighs. With the Mudra, we are sending reflexogenic feedback to the brainstem neurons in Chinmaya Bindu of the Aprakasha Bindu to focus on the middle area of the lungs. This is a message of interpersonal communication. The dynamic nature of our mind (rajas) is balanced. This practice benefits the middle section of the body and the subtle body of the Sukshma Sharira.

Adhyam Pranayama with Adhi Mudra (Adhi Means "Higher" as in Higher Section and Higher Frequency of Mind)

When adding the Hasta Adhi Mudra, place the thumb inside the other fingers and place them on the inner thighs. This gesture signifies that the supreme Self, the Atman (the thumb), is hidden in the sensory world (the other fingers). With the Mudra, we are communicating with the brainstem neurons of the Adhyam Bindu in the Aprakasha Bindu to focus on the upper area of the lungs. This is a message of transpersonal communication. The luminous nature of the mind (sattva) is awakened. This practice benefits the area of the head and neck of the body and awakens the causal body, the Karana Sharira.

Mahat Yoga Pranayama/Pranava Pranayama with Brahma Mudra (Mahat Means "Great, Grand, Complete")

When adding the Hastha Mudra, we perform the Brahma Mudra, which stimulates the Aprakasha Bindu in its totality. The Mudra is placed on the Nabhi (nābhi), the location of the psychic umbilical cord connecting us to the Great Universal Mother. The name Brahma (brāhma) is, as Swamiji teaches, "the oldest word we have in Sanskrit for breath," which is also "the word which is used for God. God is breath" (Giri, 1976, p.A-21). The fingers' position is the same as in the Adhi Mudra but here the hands are turned up towards the navel area, bringing the knuckles together with the fingers pointing upwards.

It may be interesting to notice that progression of the three mudras maps, in gesture, the teachings of Shabda Pratyahara,[9] in which we progressively bring our sense of hearing under the control of the mind. We begin the practice by bringing our sense of hearing under the control of the mind. As with Chin Mudra, we expand our listening capacity while we continue to listen deeply. Then, we begin to withdraw our senses just like we withdraw the fingers towards the palms in Chinmaya Mudra. Next, we go inside, tuning in to the inner sounds with the Adhi Mudra. Lastly, we perform the Brahma Mudra to surrender to the Divine and, with grace, to be able to tune in to the subtlest and highest of sounds, Anahata Nada.

Pranava Pranayama

There is yet another level to this practice in the teachings of Rishiculture Ashtanga (Gitananda) Yoga, the Pranava Pranayama. This Pranayama allows us to establish a direct connection with our own self and develop Swa Abhimana Bhavana (sva abhimāna bhāvana), an attitude of self-respect and self-value. Whenever we feel disconnected, alone, lonely, down, or depressed, the practice of Vibhaga Pranayama and Pranava Pranayama brings an immediate relief to our physical, emotional, mental, and spiritual health.

Swami Gitananda offers a complete instruction, which we are reproducing in full:

> An extra dimension can be added to the [Mahat Yoga] Pranayama by "thinking" the Mantrika sound associated with the appropriate lung area.

9 See Chapter 1.

> Lower breathing is governed by the sound "Aah," middle breath by the sound "Ooh," high, clavicular breath by the sound of "Mmm," while total breath, the complete union of all parts of the breathing apparatus, is controlled by the sound of "Aah… Ooh… Mmm," the Pranava Mantra AUM or OM. Think the sound "Ahh" when taking in the abdominal breath, then let out the breath with an audible "Ahh" for a longer period of time than the inspired breath. Repeat three or four times. Do the same with "Ooo" for the mid-chest and the "Mmm" for the upper breath. Conclude with a few rounds of complete breath using "AUM" in the same fashion. For the first few days, do the breath in a cycle of 1:2, that is, the outgoing breath is double the time of whatever time you chose for the in-breath. If the breath is taken for a six count, then the ratio of the outbreath is a twelve count. Try higher counts 8:16, 9:18, 10:20, and 12:24. Later, practice a 1:3 ratio, and later still, 1:4 ratio of the breath. This is called Pranava Pranayama and has great Yogic benefits as it is the first Yoga through Union of the breath that you have achieved. Extensive health benefits will also be noted and this Pranayama is an excellent Yoga Chikitsa, or breath therapy for those suffering from diseases of all types. (Giri, 1976, pp.A-23–24)

In the next chapter we will discuss how, from the Pranava AUM, all the Bija Mantras, the "seed sounds," emanate and how we can integrate them in our Chakra Sadhana (cakra sādhana) for health and healing.

Chapter 3

SACRED SOUNDS OF THE CHAKRAS

Tantra

The teachings of Dakshina Marga Tantra are an essential part of Rishiculture Ashtanga (Gitananda) Yoga and have been transmitted orally in a system of Karna (karṇa, "ear") Parampara (karṇa paramparā), a "line of Gurus," who have taught orally from the "mouth of the Guru to the ear" of the student (śiṣya) for centuries. Yogamaharishi Dr. Swami Gitananda Giri Guru Maharaj received the sacred teachings from his illustrious Guru, Swami Kanakananda Bhrigu, who received them from his Guru, Swami Vivideshananda. These were aurally received from his Guru, the Bengali saint Swami Purnananda Bhrigu, in an uninterrupted oral transmission that originated in the magnanimous teachings of Bhrigu Rishi (bhṛgu ṛṣi), one of the Sapta Rishis (saptaṛṣi). To him is attributed the composition of the *Atharvaveda* (atharvaveda), whose Yantric-Mantric-Tantric teachings include all aspects of life, from health and medicine to spirituality and astrology.

Swami Purnanada Brighu wrote 26 works (pāda), some of which were later translated into English by Sir John Woodroffe, whose pen name was Arthur Avalon.[1] The principles and practices introduced in this chapter,

1 Sir John Woodroffe (b.1865) was a British Advocate-General of Bengal and a High Court Judge who became deeply interested in Bengali Tantra, studied Sanskrit, and translated some of the classical Tantric scriptures into English, thus introducing Tantra to Great Britain and the West as early as 1913 under the pen name of Arthur Avalon. In his book *The Serpent Power: Being the ṣaṭ-cakra-nirūpaṇa and pādukā-pañcaka* (Woodroffe, 2009), published in 1922, Woodroffe translated and commented on the teachings of Swami Purnananda's *Shat Chakra Nirupana*, the "formless six energy wheels."

including the concepts of Prana, Nadi, Panchakosha (pañcakośa), Chakras, and Dhara Bija Mantras (dhara bīja mantra), may be traced back to the teachings of Swami Purnananda Brighu.[2]

Swami Gitananda Giri defined the Sanskrit term Tantra as the science of energy (tan) control (tra), a science that teaches us how to live beyond the constructs of space and time through the awareness and control of subtle psychic energies and how they manifest in our "energy body." This Pure Energy of Shakti condenses in the Tanmatras (tan, "energy"; mātra, "form"), the subtle elemental forms, called in English "the five senses," or the energies that allow us to smell, taste, touch, see, feel, and listen. At the level of cognition (jñāna), humans interact with these energies through the five organs of cognition, the Jnanendriyas, and, at the physical level, we "activate" these energies through our five organs of action, the Karmendriyas. The focus of this chapter is the process of involution from our sensorial and material reality back "hOMe" to the original source of energy through the invocation and evocation of the Dhara Bija Mantras of Chakras, psychic energy vortexes.

Prana and Pranayama

Prana is the life energy force that sustains all visible and invisible realms of manifestation, "the Supreme Spirit, the Atman, the Soul or Spirit," also referred to, in Yoga, as "The Breath of Life" (Giri, 2008, p.2). When we talk about Life, we are not simply referring to what "looks" alive to our limited senses. Even a dried leaf contains Prana, as is demonstrated by the fact that we can still make tea or cook with it. Yogamaharishi Dr. Swami Gitananda Giri teaches that the word Prana:

> is derived from the compounding of "Pra"—"self-existence, prior existence, prior to"; and "Ana"—"cells, conglomerates, units, food." Therefore, Prana means that which existed before anything was created, yet is present in all things that are manifested or created. (Giri, 2008, p.3)

---

2 These teachings are advanced and require a direct transmission from Guru to Shishya (śiṣya), a committed student, and, therefore, will only be introduced in this chapter with the goal of clarifying some of these concepts that, over the last two decades, especially in English translations of "New Age" disseminations, have been corrupted with misinformation and rough approximations. If you are interested in learning more and going deeper in the practices, please contact the authors to learn about upcoming training programs.

Once Prana enters our body it is used for various physiological functions and manifests through five major Vital Airs, the Pancha Prana Vayus (pañca prāṇa vāyu), and five minor Vital Airs, the Upa Prana Vayus (upa prāṇa vāyu). Pranayama is the "Science of Breath," "the Control of the Vital Force (Prana) in the air we breathe. ... Prana is the Divine Mother Energy, the Universal Creative Power, and Ayaama means 'controlled expansion' or 'science of control'" (Giri, 2008, p.14).

The Nadis

In the human body, Prana flows in three ways (Giri, 2008, p.7):

- As Prana Vayu (prāṇa vāyu), it moves like "an airflow."
- As Prana Vahaka (prāṇa vāhaka), it moves as impulses caroming from neural cell to cell.
- As Prana Vahana (prāṇa vāhana), it oozes as fluid through the walls of cells and tissues.

Prana moves through subtle energy channels called Nadi, a Sanskrit term that is used to describe a "vein" or a "channel" and also "a flow." "The term Nadi," Swamiji teaches, "may describe blood or lymph flow but in Adhyatmika Yoga, the higher aspects of Yoga, the term Nadi is always used to describe the channel through which Prana and other higher energies flow into Chakras and Bindus" (Giri, 1976, p.A-46). There are thousands of "energy channels" in our psychic body. Classical Yoga scriptures list 72,000 Nadis, and many of them take the names from Indian rivers.

The three main channels are the Pingala Nadi, the "right channel," the Ida Nadi, the "left channel," and the Sushumna Nadi, the "central channel," which, flowing from beyond the bottom of the spine and beyond the top of the skull, creates an axial pathway (mokṣa mārga) for Prana to flow in the highest experience of liberation through the realization of immortality.[3] As Georg Feuerstein writes, the name Sushumna Nadi may be translated as

3 As Swamiji teaches, this ascension and liberation can only occur if one has prepared physically, emotionally, and mentally through the steady practice of the preliminary and foundational steps of Yoga, the Bahiranga Yoga (bahiraṅga yoga) of Yama, Niyama, Asana, Pranayama, and Pratyahara.

"most gracious current," because it is the "royal road to freedom" (Feuerstein, 1998, p.162).

Pingala is related to the sun (sūrya) and to gold, and it is a channel for the energy of activation, warmth, and excitation. Its energetic flow regulates the sympathetic nervous system and the functions of the left hemisphere. Ida is related to the moon (candra) and to silver, and it is a channel for the energy of magnetism, cooling off, and relaxation. Its energetic flow regulates the parasympathetic nervous system and the functions of the right hemisphere. Sushumna, as the main and central energy channel, allows for an integrated convergence of the other two.

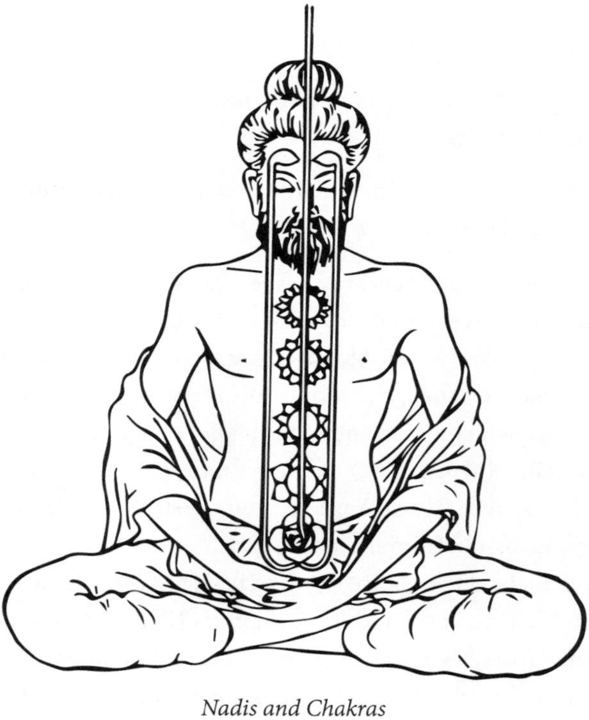

Nadis and Chakras

Inside the Sushumna is Chitra (citrā), a smaller subtle channel connecting to the energetic area on the top of the skull called the Brahmarandhra, the skull's anterior fontanelle, from which Prana leaves the body of Yogis[4] at the time of

4 The term Yogi is used here to define serious and assiduous practitioners, men and women, of Yoga who have reached a state of Self-realization.

death. The three Nadis originate in an "energy bulb" in the area at the bottom of the spine, the Kanda (kanda) at Muladhara Chakra (mūlādhāra cakra), the Root Energy Center, where they are joined together as "triple-braided yoke," Yukta Triveni (yukta triveṇī). They free themselves of the union with the other two at the brow center, the Third Eye at Ajna Chakra, Mukta Triveni (mukta triveṇī).

The Panchakoshas

The *Taittirya Upanishad* (taittirīyopaniṣad), one of the primary *Upanishads* and part of the *Krishna Yajur Veda*, contains a very important teaching on the "five bodies," the five Pranic sheaths (pañcakośa) that constitute and sustain our human experience. Most likely written down from oral transmission around the 6th century BCE, it consists of three parts called Valli, a term that refers to the "growth of a vine," a metaphor for the life force of the teachings they contain. The second Valli, the Brahmananda Valli (brahmānanda valli), consists of ten verses, and it teaches that human evolution, as part of the evolution of the Universe, derives from Brahman, a Cosmic Intelligence. Yoga, Union with that Supreme Consciousness, is a process of involution, of going "back" to the Source. To achieve this, we need to realize that we are made of several energy bodies, from the grossest material physical body to the most refined body of bliss, and that we need to resolve each body's existence into the one it evolved from. The five bodies, or "sheaths," are:

- Annamaya Kosha (annamayakośa): the force of anatomical existence, sustained and maintained by apparently solid matter (Anna)
- Pranamaya Kosha (prāṇamayakośa): the force of physiological existence, sustained and maintained by individual energy (Prana)
- Manomaya Kosha (manomayakośa): the force of psychological existence, sustained and maintained by the mind (Manas)
- Vijnanamaya Kosha (vijñānamayakośa): the force of intellectual existence, sustained and maintained by the intellect of the Higher Mind (Buddhi)
- Anandamaya Kosha (ānandamayakośa): the force of cosmic existence, sustained and maintained by bliss (Ananda).

The Koshas are always present and active, as they are part of our existence. They are "energy structures" that surround each other. For example, the Pranamaya Kosha, or "body of Prana," is both inside the physical body, in the flow of nervous impulses and fluids, and surrounding the physical body, in our overall emotional communication with what is "outside" of us. In a similar way, the sheath of mind, the Manomaya Kosha, is the subconscious and conscious intelligence that activates our cells to behave in a specific way and, similarly, it is an intelligence that allows us to perceive external reality. Koshas expand outwards and inwards. Each one of our cells, for example, has five Koshas:

- Annamaya Kosha: the cell's structural existence
- Pranamaya Kosha: the cell's functional mechanisms
- Manomaya Kosha: the cellular memory
- Vijnanamaya Kosha: the cell's intelligent feedback mechanisms
- Anandamaya Kosha: the cell's systemic interactivity.

What holds the bodies together is Prana. While a conscious and dynamic integration of all the layers of existence results in Self-knowledge (to be "at ease" with the awareness of Self), a disassociation of the sheaths will result in a variety of psychosomatic disorders (the experience of dis-ease of the self). As Swami Gitananda teaches:

> whenever the Prana is inhibited by wrong emotions, false thoughts or improper living habits, then Prana Nara ensues. The Koshas are forced apart, creating psychic disassociation. Visible manifestations of Prana Nara are psychotic and neurotic tendencies as well as those conditions termed psychosomatic disorders. (Giri, 2008, p.11)

It is therefore of vital importance to become aware of the Koshas and to harmonize them through serious practices. In Chapter 2 we detailed the Vibhaga and Pranava Pranayama as excellent practices to harmonize the various sections of the lungs, parts of the brain, areas of the body, dimensions of the mind, and beyond. In this chapter, we introduce the teachings on the Chakras Dhara Bija Mantras and Gayatri Mantras (gāyatrī mantra) that express the energetic flows of the Chakras to tune in and enjoy each center's qualities and look at how they benefit our psychosomatic health and healing.

The Chakras

One of the ways in which the cosmic life force of Prana seems to flow is in vortices and whirlpools. Spirals can be observed everywhere in nature—from the movement of galaxies, helixes of our DNA, ocean tides, tornadoes, and water flowing down our sinkholes, to the shape of our fingerprints, seashells, sunflower seeds, and crystal formations. Yogamaharishi Dr. Swami Gitananda Giri teaches that, in holding the five bodies together, Prana "sets up great vortexes of energy in certain parts of the nervous system, creating Psychic Centers, which are called Chakras (lit. wheels) or Padmas (lit. lotuses)" (Giri, 2008, p.20). When the centers are described for their function, as energy vortexes, they are called Chakras; when they are described structurally, by number of petals, they are called Padmas (padma), "lotuses."[5] Each center has a number of energy flows depicted as the petals of a lotus flower.

In the teachings of our Parampara, we are made aware of Twelve Chakras (dvādaśa cakrani): six lower Chakras (ṣaṭ cakra) referred to as Pinda Chakras (piṇḍa, "individuality"), the centers that enable us to experience life as individuals, and six higher Chakras, called the Mahakarana Chakras, the great Causal Centers, also referred to as Anda Chakras (aṇḍa, "egg"), centers of the Cosmic "Egg" Body Chakras. Pinda Chakras correspond to six main cerebrospinal areas in our bodies, their major nerve plexuses and endocrine glands, organs, and body parts, as well as emotional qualities. There are also "minor chakras" corresponding to each joint of the body. Dr. Ananda describes the Chakras as "the energy Matrix that opens us up to the Infinite Potential that lies within us. They help us understand who we are, what we are and how we are connected to this Cosmos. ... They are like energy transformers for the psychic energy" (Bhavanani, 2022).

Chakras are not located in the body, and they are not a gland or a nervous plexus; rather, they manifest in the nervous and glandular systems as an "activated energy flow" (Giri, 1976, p.A-46). The psychic pathways of the Pinda Chakras vibrate in the energy body of Pranamaya Kosha, and they are fully manifest in the Anandamaya Kosha. The Cosmic energies of the higher six Anda Chakras are, as Swamiji says, "incorrectly lumped together" and called Sahasrara Chakra (sahasrāra cakra), or the "seventh Chakra." They are our connection to the ultimate reality and are reflected in the lower six chakras,

5 In the teachings of Swami Gitananda, the term Padma is only used for the Pinda Chakras and not for the Anda Chakras.

correlated with our individual existence in its sensual manifestation. What makes us conscious and thriving human beings are the Shat Anda Chakras, the energies of the Universe, which infuse the Shat Pinda Chakras with Pranic energy. The macrocosm, Brahmanda (brahmāṇḍa), and the microcosm, Pindam (piṇḍam), coincide, as taught in this Mantra, which may be uttered as a Japa to remind us of the connectivity between our Pinda and Anda Chakras:

यत् पिण्डे तत् ब्रह्माण्डे
यत् ब्रह्माण्डे तत् पिण्डे

yat piṇḍe tat brahmāṇḍe
yat brahmāṇḍe tat piṇḍe

That which is in the individual microcosm is in the whole cosmos.
That which is in the macrocosm is in the individual.

The "above and below" are truly One. The sense of separation is spiritual ignorance, Avidya (avidyā). From the Ultimate Reality of Parama-Shiva (parama śiva), which consists of an integration of Pure Consciousness, Shiva, and Pure Energy, Shakti, the sensorial world manifests in progressive stages of condensation resulting in Maya, the "illusion of reality" as we perceive and conceive it through our senses, including the sixth sense of intellect and mind. Maya is our worldly day-to-day reality in which the differentiation of Spirit (puruṣa) and Matter (prakṛti) manifest. In Prakriti, the three qualities of the Gunas coexist: Tamas (tamas), inertia and indolence; Rajas (rajas), dynamism and activity; Satwa (satva), luminosity and purity. When the Gunas are in a perfect state of equilibrium, Prakriti is unmanifested and in a state of quiet potentiality. In the human cycles of reincarnation, however, due to the fruits of past actions (karma), the Gunas are in a state of dynamic "con-fusion." The process of their imbalance generates the Tattwas (tattva), principles that manifest and sustain the reality we live in. This is the process of evolution from All that is, Purusha (puruṣa), to our individualized experience of being:

Purusha ~ Prakriti

⇩

Mahat (buddhi): intellect

⇩

Ahamkara (ahaṃkāra): ego; "I" identity

⇩

Manas (manas): mind; cognition through sensorial perception

⇩

Jnanendriyas: Cognitive Senses
Ears, śrotra
Skin, tvac
Eyes, cakṣus
Tongue, rasanā
Nose, ghrāṇa

⇩

Karmendriyas: Action Instruments
Speech and Sense of Communication, vāk
Genitals and Sense of Reproduction, upastha
Anus and Sense of Excretion, pāyu
Hands and Sense of Dexterity, pāṇi
Feet and Sense of Locomotion, pāda

⇩

Tanmatras: The Five Subtle Elements
Sound, śabda
Touch, sparśa
Form, rūpa
Taste, rasa
Smell, gandha

⇩

Mahabhuta (pañca mahābhūta): The Five "Gross" Elements
Ether, and the Ethereal State, ākāśa
Air and the Gaseous State, vāyu
Fire and the Thermal State, tejas
Water and the Liquid State, apas
Earth and the Solid State, pṛthivī

The Twelve Chakras follow this evolutionary process from the subtlest to the denser, from the manifestation of Buddhi down to the experience of dense earth. When understood in this way, the 12th Chakra of Mokshana Chakra becomes the first to manifest and, vice versa, the first Chakra of Muladhara is the last of the 12 to condense. However, in our process of involution from density to luminosity, from con-fusion with what is transitory to the realization of That which is eternal, from bondage to attachment to freedom, Muladhara is numbered as the "first Chakra" because it is our "first step" back "hOMe."

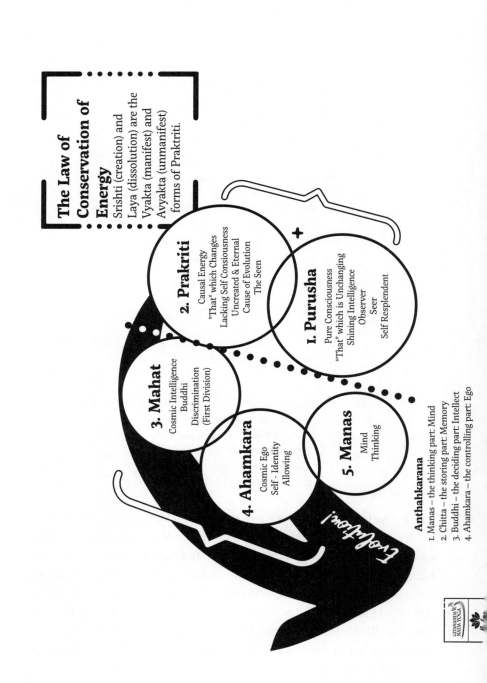

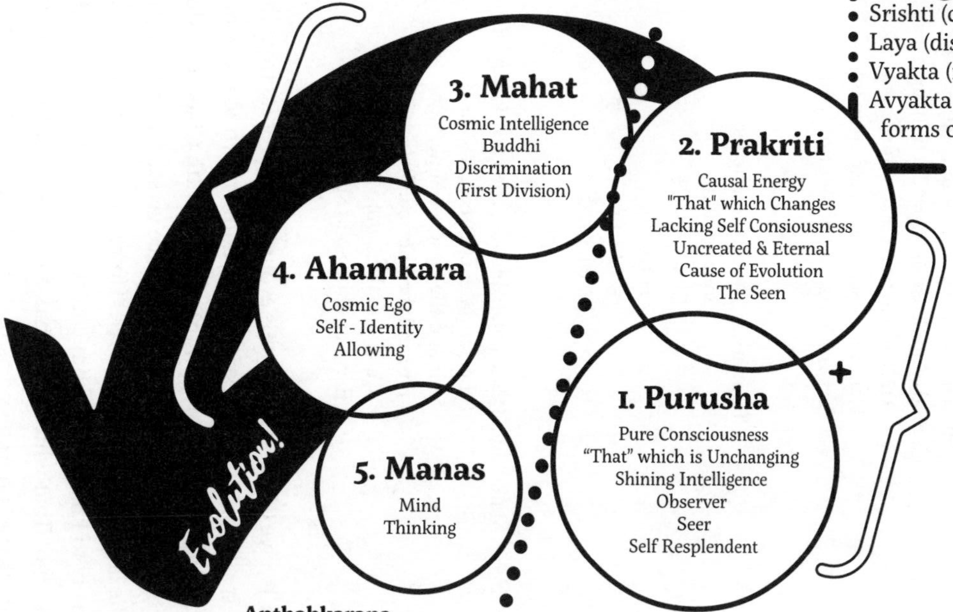

The Law of Conservation of Energy

Srishti (creation) and Laya (dissolution) are the Vyakta (manifest) and Avyakta (unmanifest) forms of Praktriti.

Anthahkarana

1. Manas – the thinking part: Mind
2. Chitta – the storing part: Memory
3. Buddhi – the deciding part: Intellect
4. Ahamkara – the controlling part: Ego

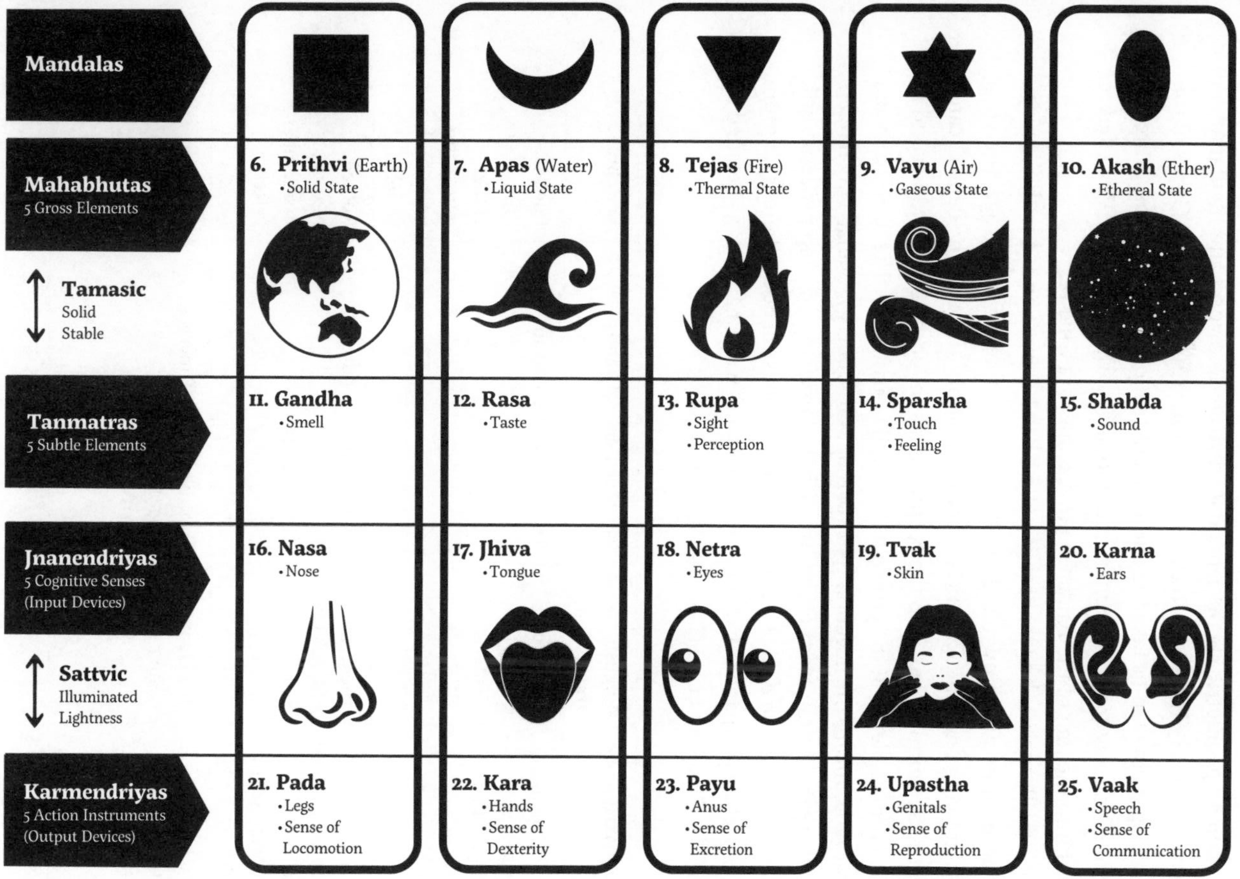

Evolution of Tattwas

A color version of this image can be downloaded from uk.singingdragon.com/catalogue/book/9781839974502.

The practices that Rishiculture Ashtanga Yoga assigns to each Chakra, from postures (āsana), to specific patterns of breathing (prāṇāyāma), to concentration on geometric shapes (maṇḍala dhāraṇa), to vocal and mental utterances (mantra), have been transmitted uninterruptedly by the Gurus of the Parampara to help us take the energy from the lower six Chakras, center by center, starting from Muladhara and moving all the way up to Ajna Chakra and into the first of the Anda Chakras, Sahasrara Chakra.

The Prana in the Chakras is called Vana (vāṇa) and it is this energy that must be withdrawn and lifted in the practices of Laya Yoga, the yoga of "drawing back the Cosmic energy of creation" through the central canal of the Sushumna Nadi into the corpus callosum of the brain and beyond in the coronal plexus at the crown of the skull (Giri, 1984). The term Nir-vana (nirvāṇa) means the negation "Nir" of that Pranic energy "Vana," which refers to its reabsorption from each lower Chakra in a step-by-step process until, once we reach the Anda Chakras beyond the physical body, there is no more form left, Ni-rupana (nirūpaṇa). Here are the Twelve Chakras as detailed by Swami Gitananda Giri (Giri, 1976, pp.A-46–48):

Sanskrit name	**English translation**	**Nerve center**	**Gland**	**Vertebrae**
1. Muladhara Chakra (mūlādhāra cakra)	The Root Support Center	Sacral plexus	Gonads	Rooted at the junction of the fourth and fifth sacral vertebrae
2. Swadhishthana Chakra (svādhiṣṭhāna cakra)	The Center of One's Own Self	Hypo-gastric plexus or pelvic plexus	Adrenals	Rooted near the first lumbar vertebra
3. Manipura Chakra (maṇipūra cakra)	The Gem City Center	Solar plexus or gastric plexus	Pancreas	Rooted at the eighth thoracic or dorsal vertebra

4. Anahata Chakra (anāhata cakra)	The Center of Unstruck Sound	Cardiac plexus	Thymus	Rooted near the seventh cervical vertebra
5. Vishuddha Chakra (viśuddha cakra)	The Center of Great Purity	Pharyngeal plexus	Thyroid and parathyroids	Rooted near the third cervical vertebra
6. Ajna Chakra (ajña cakra)	The Center of Revelation	Cavernous plexus	Pituitary gland	Above the midpoint between the eyebrows
7. Sahasrara Chakra (sahasrāra cakra)	The Center of the Thousand-Petalled Lotus	Coronal plexus	Pineal gland	Top of the head
8. Narayanana Chakra (nārāyaṇana cakra)	The Center of the Breath of Substance		Hypothalamus	Outside of the left ear Cerebellum
9. Brahmanana Chakra (brahmaṇana cakra)	The Center of the Breath of Creativeness		Thalamus	Outside of the right ear Cerebrum
10. Trikuti Chakra (trikūṭi cakra)	The Pyramidal Center		Pyramidal, extra pyramidal area of the brain	Above the head
11. Swaminana Chakra (svāmīṇana cakra)	The Breath of the Master Center or Guru Chakra		Prefrontal cortex	Above the head, left
12. Mokshana/ Mukti Chakra (mokṣana cakra)	The Center of Spiritual Freedom		Arachnoid membrane	Above the head, right

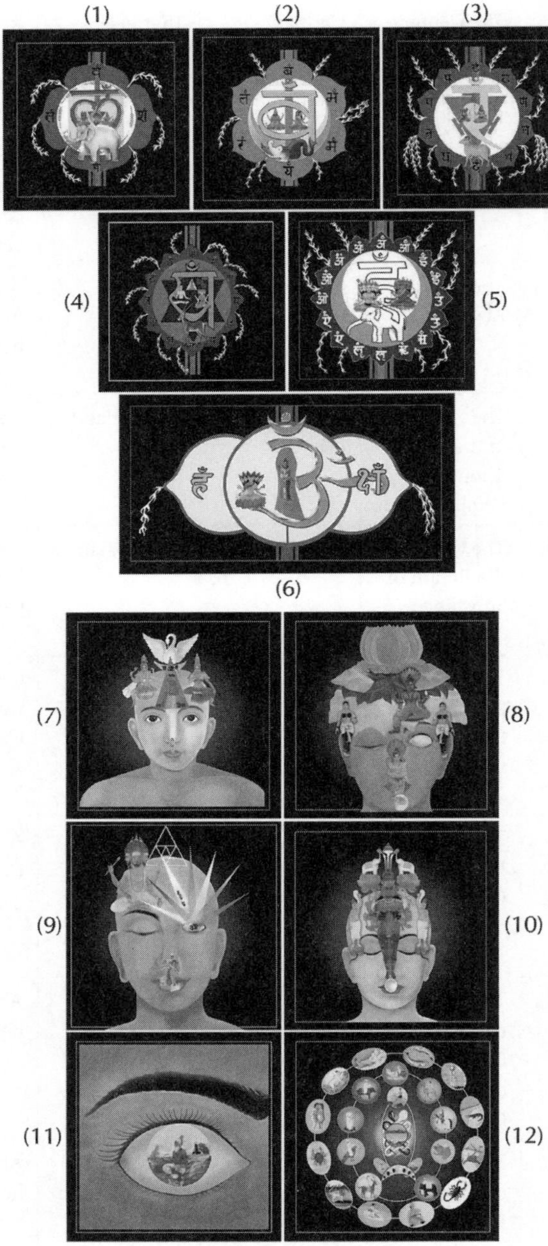

Pinda Chakras/Anda Chakras
A color version of this image can be downloaded from uk.singingdragon.com/catalogue/book/9781839974502.

Above Sahasrara Chakra, the other five Anda Chakras end with "ana," referring to the "breath of," such as, for example, Narayanana Chakra, "the Breath of Vishnu." These are "universal Chakras" rather than individual centers and are arranged as a halo around the area of our head rather than in a level-by-level series of spirals:

- Narayanana Chakra is the eighth chakra of 12, and is related to the energy of manifestation, birth, and conservation.
- The next one, number nine, is the Brahmananda Chakra, related to the higher energy of universal creativity and the ability to tap into it.
- Trikuti Chakra is number ten, the "escape center," where the Prana enters and "leaves" the body.[6]
- The 11th chakra is the Swaminana Chakra. There is an understanding of the Swa (sva), the self, at a higher level, when and where the individual self is giving over to the universal higher Self. This is the Swami, somebody who has truly realized the nature of the Self.
- Muktana is the highest and fastest of the energy centers. This Chakra is related to the concepts of Mukhti and Moksha, terms that refer to liberation, enlightenment, and Kaivalya (kaivalya), final freedom from bondage.

Pinda Chakras

Each of the Pinda Chakras, as well as Sahasrara Chakra, has a correspondence with a nervous plexus and a gland. The lower five centers also correspond to a subtle element (tanmātrā), a "great" element (mahābhūta), a sense organ (jñānendriya), an organ of action, and a Prana Vayu (life giving winds).

6 Gitananda Yoga practices include several concentration techniques to learn how to bring the energy of Prana beyond the head so that, at the time of death, by exhaling the last breath through the Trikuti Bindu and Chakra, one may "escape" the cycle of birth, death, and rebirth and become a liberated soul.

	Pinda Chakras Lower (Somatic) Vortices of Energy	**Body Root** Glands & Plexii (Anamaya)	**Dala (Petals)** Major Energy Flow	**Dhara Bija** Seed Sound (Initiates universal harmonization)	**Mandalas**
Ajna	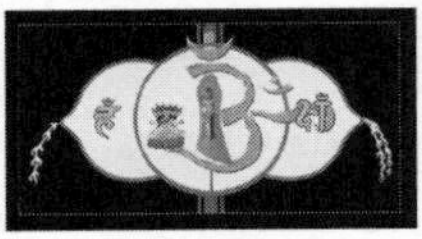	**Intuition** • Nasion between Eyes • Pituitary Gland • Cavernous Plexus	**2**	A + ng (Aum) ॐ	
Vishuddha	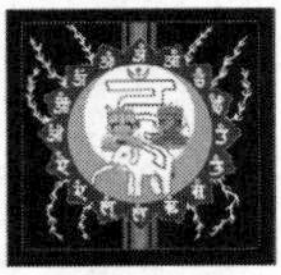	**Great Purity** • Throat Region • Thyroid & Para-Thyroid Glands • Pharyngeal Plexus	**16**	Ha + ng हं	
Anahata	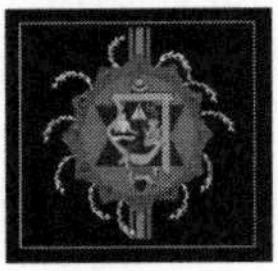	**Unstruck Sound** • Heart Region • Thymus • Cardiac Plexus	**12**	Ya + ng यं	
Manipura	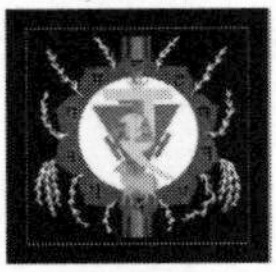	**Gem City** • Navel Region • Pancreas (Endocrine) & Liver • Solar Plexus	**10**	Ra + ng रं	
Swadhisthana	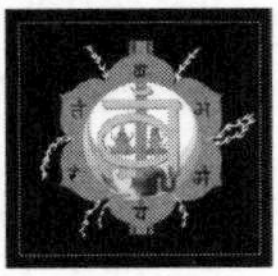	**One's Own Abode** • Pelvic Region • Adrenal Glands • Hypogastric Plexus	**6**	Va + ng वं	
Muladhara	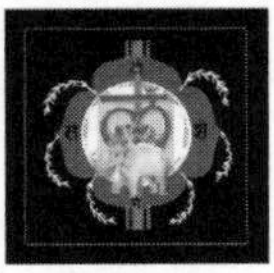	**Root Support** • Base of Spine (Coccyx) • Gonads (Testes & Ovaries) • Sacral Plexus	**4**	La + ng लं	

Pinda Chakras, Bija, and Tattwas

A color version of this image can be downloaded from uk.singingdragon.com/catalogue/book/9781839974502.

Mahabhutas 5 Gross Elements	**Tanmatras** 5 Subtle Elements	**Jnanendriyas** 5 Cognitive Senses (Input Devices)	**Karmendriyas** 5 Action Instruments (Output Devices)	**Qualities**	**Hatha Yoga** Asana for a Healthy Spine
					• Padmasana in Shirsha Asana • Kapala Asana
Akash • Ethereal State 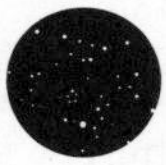	**Shabda** • Sound	**Karna** • Ears 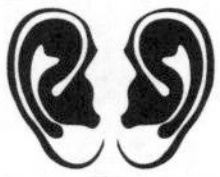	**Vaak** • Speech • Sense of Communication	• Freedom • Communication • Empathy	• Sarvanga Asana
Vayu • Gaseous State 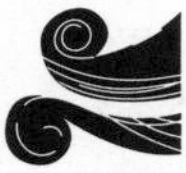	**Sparsha** • Touch • Feeling	**Tvak** • Skin 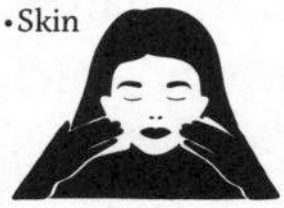	**Upastha** • Genitals • Sense of Reproduction	• Compassion • Tolerance • Understanding	• Ardha Matsyendrasana Brahmadanda Asana • Vakra Asana • Gomukha Asana
Tejas • Thermal State 	**Rupa** • Sight • Perception	**Netra** • Eyes 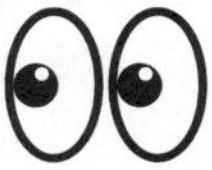	**Payu** • Anus • Sense of Excretion	• Power • Passion • Motivation	• Dharmika Asana
Apas • Liquid State 	**Rasa** • Taste	**Jhiva** • Tongue 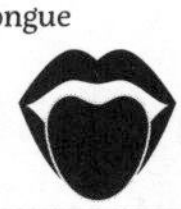	**Kara** • Hands • Sense of Dexterity	• Flexibility • Diplomacy • Equanimity	• Supta Vajra Asana • Matsya Asana
Prithvi • Solid State 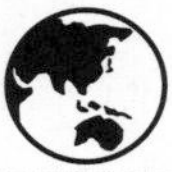	**Gandha** • Smell	**Nasa** • Nose 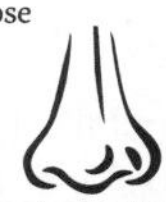	**Pada** • Legs • Sense of Locomotion	• Integration • Solidarity • Cohesiveness	• Vajra Asana • Sukha Asana • Siddha Asana • Padma Asana

The Pinda Chakras are vortices that spiral clockwise around the Brahmadanda (brahmadaṇḍa), "the Staff of God," located, physically, around our spine. Our vertebral column is an antenna that, at the metaphysical level, receives "cosmic energy," while at the physical level, it functions as the medium through which all the neurological activities happen.

"Cosmic energy," taught Swami Gitananda, "activates at least four of the twelve major Chakras with the 'first breath of life'" (Giri, 1976, p.A-46). At every birth, the higher three centers, namely Mokshana, Swaminana, and Trikuti Chakras, are open for everyone. Then, according to the time, place, and circumstances of birth, Prana is funneled into our physical, physiological, emotional, and mental bodies through a "psychic umbilical cord"[7] and, from here, it activates one of the Chakras related to our "birth path," the Dharma Marga (dharma mārga).[8] This becomes the primary center for our existence in this lifetime because it points to our Dharma, our capacity to abide by the "Cosmic Law." As Pujya Ammaji often teaches, "Dharma implies that one willfully chooses to perform the right action, at the right moment in the right manner, no matter how much personal sacrifice such an action may entail." Learning which Dharma Marga we walk on in our incarnation and how to "work" with the relative Chakra contributes to our psychosomatic well-being.

In some of the Hindu scriptures the Divine is portrayed as having many heads, arms, eyes, and feet. That is not what God is. What this means is that every one of our heads is a head of the Divine, so that the Divine may think through us; our eyes are the eyes of the Divine, so that the Divine may see through us; our hands are the hands of the Divine, so that the Divine may work through us; our feet are the feet of the Divine, so that the Divine may move through us.

The Sahasrara Chakra has a physical correlation in the pineal gland that enables us to understand the difference between darkness and light at the physical, emotional, mental, and spiritual levels. This is our true Third Eye,

7 This psychic umbilical cord corresponds to the umbilical button at the navel but it is slightly higher, in the diaphragmatic area of the "solar plexus."

8 Dharma Marga is the definition of a "birth path" in the numerological system of Yantra. One's "birth path" is one digit that is obtained by summing all the digits of our birthday together. There are nine Dharma Margas; therefore the first five Chakras are "assigned" as a path at birth, from one, Muladhara, to nine, Brahmanana (Giri, 1995). These teachings are available through online courses by Yogacharya Dr. Ananda Balayogi Bhavanani.

a center that regulates our inner rhythms so that we attune ourselves to the Cosmos in which we are living and experience "health" and "harmony." A reconnection with all energies occurs in this center.

Dhara Bija Mantra Sadhana

Bija Mantra Sadhana is a gem of the Rishiculture Ashtanga Yoga teachings, a wonderful technology drawn from our Tantric lineage. The teachings on the Chakras are Tantric in nature and the study of Mantra is at the heart of the *Atharvaveda*. Akshara (akṣara) in Sanskrit refers to that which cannot be broken down into smaller units, the unbreakable. Each of the phonemes of Samskrita (saṃskṛta), the Sanskrit alphabet, is an Akshara; whether it be the Swara (svara), a vowel, or the Viajnana (vyañjana), consonant, each is a single unit of sound. Each of the Chakras has its own key sound, the Bijaksharas (bījākṣara), which acts like a password to awaken the infinite potential that lies in each one of us.

Bija Mantras are very high vibrations that, while being part of Sanskrit phonemes as one-syllable sounds, are free of linguistic specification. Bija Mantras are essential sounds whose meaning is the vibration itself and not an external point of reference. They are the condensation of sound emanating from the pure Cosmic vibration of Para-Vac. If we accept a simile between the vibration of the Pranava AUM and that of the Big Bang, then the phonemes of the Sanskrit alphabet are like galaxies condensing from that primal manifestation. Slowly, as it becomes denser, this sonic energy manifests the language as we use it in our daily speech of Vaikhari Vac.[9]

Bija is a seed of infinite potential (Ja means "to give birth"), a seed that has the capacity to give birth to what seems like infinity. What enables the potential that is hidden in the seed, the latent potential to manifest, is Prana, the life force. A seed needs to have life force. When we plant a seed, we need to have the wisdom, Viveka, to plant it in fertile soil, to nourish it, and to take care of it. We began our lifetime from a seed from the father, the sperm, the smallest single cell, and the ovum from the mother, the largest single cell. Nature is the potential that lies in that seed and nurture is the mindfulness that enables that potential to manifest and become an actuality.

9 For the four levels of Vac, see Chapter 1.

The Dhara Bija Mantras for the Pinda Chakras and the Sahasrara Chakra are:

- Lang (laṃ) for Muladhara
- Vang (vaṃ) for Swadhishthana
- Rang (raṃ) for Manipura
- Yang (yaṃ) for Anahata
- Hang (haṃ) for Vishuddha
- Ang (aṃ) for Ajna
- Aum (oṃ) for Sahasrara.[10]

LA, VA, RA, YA, HA, A are all phonemes of the Sanskrit alphabet[11] that have been "activated" by the sound of the Anuswara, a cerebro-nasal tone (NG), typically transliterated by a dot over the M, as in Oṁ, and, in Tantra, by the Chandra Bindu, depicted as a point over a crescent, the "moon point" ँ. This "nasal twang" is what differentiates the sound of Bija Mantras from the sound of Sanskrit letters. Once we reach Sahasrara Chakra, we intone the Pranava Mantra AUM, which contains the vibration of the combined Anda Chakras and the Pinda Chakras and 50 Sanskrit phonemes including the sound of Ksha-ng (kṣaṃ).[12]

Through dedicated and sincere Chakra Bija Mantra Sadhana, we become aware of the vibratory essence of the Chakras and learn to relax as we "attune" ourselves to the highest vibration of the Self, of Brahman, of Para-Nada. First, we study the principles and philosophical precepts; then, when we are ready to practice, we "sit up"[13] and connect with the flows of Prana in our bodies

10 In some traditions, the Pranava Oṁ is located in the area of Ajna Chakra at the mid-brow center.

11 LA, VA, RA, YA are semivowels; HA is an aspirate guttural consonant; A is a guttural vowel. AUM is the sum of all sounds of the Varnamala.

12 In the more advanced practices of Mantra Laya, the 50 phonemes of the Sanskrit alphabet, intoned as the Chakra Dala Bija Mantras, are repeated 20 times for a total of 1000 sounds whose vibrations culminate in the Pranava AUM and are "held in Dharana" in the Thousand-Petalled Lotus of Sahasrara Chakra.

13 Ammaji always reminds us that in Yoga we "sit up" rather than "sit down." This implies choosing postures that help us keep our spine vertically aligned, keep our limbs calm and collected in specific Asanas and Mudras, and regulate our breathing patterns.

by regulating our breathing cycles. We "invoke" each Bija Mantra by thinking about its sound and then "evoke" it by uttering it out loud. As we utter the sound, the inverse process begins to unfold. We inhale and, as we exhale, while keeping our mind focused on the Chakra's qualities and energies, we produce the sound.

Taking the example of the Dhara Bija Lang for Muladhara Chakra (see the chart below), we begin with the uttered sound of LA, imagining that it emanates from the center of our body, from the area that corresponds to it—in this case, the sacral plexus of the sacral region. The sound waves move out of our body in a 360-degree pattern, like the ripple effect of waves when we drop a stone at the center of a calm pond. LA is like a mallet striking a bell and like the stone that plunges in the still waters. To potentiate it, we add the cerebro-nasal -ng sound produced by turning the tip of the tongue up to touch the midpoint between the soft and hard palate. While we do this, we begin to reabsorb the sound back into the center of our bodies, and once it returns to the point where LA originated, it becomes LAM, whose after-tone is rippling out to the causal plane, into the transcendental. We cannot "make" that transcendental sound with our voice. The personality has to be discarded for the universality to manifest. In the representation below, we attempt to offer a clarification on the progress of involution from the "gross" utterance of a Mantra to its "acoustic sublimation" into silence.

La	Lang	Lam	
Vaikhari	Madhyama	Pashyanti Para	
Interpersonal	**Intrapersonal**	**Transpersonal**	
Pratyahara	Dharana	Dhyana	Samadhi
Ahata Nada		Anahata Nada	

This process of reabsorption is even more fully explored in the practice of Mantra Laya in which all of the Sanskrit phonemes are invoked as the Dala Bija Mantras (dala bīja mantra), the sounds of each Chakra's petals.[14] It is

14 These teachings come from an oral tradition, from the mouth of the Guru to the ear of the student, in an uninterrupted transmission of Karna (ear) Parampara (lineage). The authors chose to share only the practices of Dhara Bija Mantra Sadhana in the book, with the hope that sincere aspirants may want to learn the more advanced practices of Nada Yoga directly from Dr. Ananda and from qualified Mentors of Rishiculture Ashtanga (Gitananda) Yoga.

as if we could imagine our planetary system, all of the suns in our galaxies, and all galaxies becoming reabsorbed into the grand explosion of the Big Bang—at an acoustic level.

Maharishi Patanjali, in the second Pada of the *Yoga Sutra*, Sadhana Pada, describes a similar process of "reversing" the vibrations of the Kleshas into the mind as a form of involution back to the Source, from gross to inaudible, from subtle to causal:

> [II:10]
>
> ते प्रतिप्रसवहेयाः सूक्ष्माः ॥ १० ॥
>
> te pratiprasava-heyāḥ sūkṣmāḥ
>
> *One must go against the very subtle source of these afflictions [if they are to be eradicated]* (Bhavanani, 2011a, p.123).

The Chakra Bija Mantra Sadhana is, in this sense, a form of Pratyahara, the withdrawal of the senses after their full expansion. The Mantras Lang, Vang, Rang, Yang, Hang, Ang, Om, all pronounced with the Anuswara, create a momentum for this propulsion of energy reabsorption. Their resonance is satisfying at the physical and physiological level (Tamas), for the energy they produce (Rajas), and for the silence they create in the mind (Satvas).

Dr. Ananda describes three levels of Mantra Sadhana and the importance of a process of concentration, meditation, and absorption (saṃyama) to "attune" to a Mantra:

> The first layer is where we write a sound out. We write the Sanskrit phoneme of the Bija Mantra for Muladhara Chakra "Lang," for example. The second level is where we chant the sound, making it audible. The third level is where, without producing it externally, we listen to the sound internally, in the mind. When we are able to go from the written to the spoken and above, we are able to channel the energy of the mind. … It is very essential that the mind remains focused when we do these practices. If I chant the mantra while focusing on something completely different, the power of the chant won't be activated. (Bhavanani and Biagi, 2013, p.7)

When sound is made with focused attention and repeated with purity of sentiments, we summon an intensity that turns matter into pure energy.

In this sense, the power of intent is as important as "good pronunciation":

> One of the most important aspects of Nada is not only making the sound but also where we are focusing the sound. As an example: the sunlight is everywhere but when we take a lens and focus it, it becomes a beam and its effect is much more powerful. Similarly, sounds are all around us: mantras are its lenses. (Bhavanani and Biagi, 2013, pp.7–8)

We begin at the lips, with the dental Lang in Muladhara Chakra and the labial Vang in Swadhishthana. Then we travel back inside our oral cavity, with the high cerebral articulation of the sound of Rang in Manipura, then travel towards the back of the throat with the articulation of the palatal Yang in Anahata, and then come to the lowest point of resonance, the aspirant guttural Hang of Vishuddha and the guttural vowel of Ang of Ajna Chakra. Finally, when we invoke the Pranava AUM in Sahasrara Chakra, we travel "back hOMe" from the guttural to the labial to the nasal and the cerebral.[15]

Chakra Devata Gayatri Mantras

Dhara and Dala Bija Mantras are Nirguna Mantras, which means that they are "beyond the gunas," beyond attributes such as adjectives related to sensorial specificity. There are also Nirguna Bija Mantras that are vibrating with the energy of specific deities (devatā), such as Gaṃ for Lord Ganesha. All Hindu divinities have a Beejakshara (bīja akṣara) that corresponds to them as well as a Gayatri Mantra that corresponds to the Chakra they preside over. In each Chakra "dwells" deities—masculine/feminine energy manifestations—who protect and sustain the energy of that psychic center. The following Devata are "assigned" to the Pinda Chakras with a Tantric Shakti, a feminine deity:

- Muladhara Chakra: Lord Ganesha (gaṇeśa)/Dakini (ḍākinī)
- Swadhishthana Chakra: Lord Brahma/Rakini (rākinī)
- Manipura Chakra: Lord Vishnu/Lakini (lākinī)

15 See the section "A Note on Sanskrit" at the start of this book for Sanskrit pronunciation and Chapter 2 for an elucidation of the concept and practice of vocal articulation in Pranava AUM Mantra Sadhana.

- Anahata Chakra: Lord Shiva as Rudra (rudra)/Kakini (kākinī)
- Vishuddha Chakra: Lord Shiva/Shakini (sākinī)
- Ajna Chakra: Paramshiva (paramśiva)/Hakini (hākinī).

For each Chakra, we intone a Gayatri Mantra to concentrate, meditate, and become one with its related Devata.[16] The original Gayatri Mantra can be traced back to the *Rigveda* (3.62.10). It is a Mantra of 24 syllables (eight syllables in three lines), an invocation to the benevolent Light of Savitur, the Sun, both as our solar system's star and as the Highest Light of Divinity. This Mantra was received by the Brahma Rishi Vishvamitra (viśvāmitra), to "ease the pain and suffering of humanity," and has hence been transmitted from generation to generation all the way to us.

ॐ
तत्सवितुर्वरेण्यं
भर्गो देवस्य धीमहि
धियो यो नः प्रचोदयात् ।
ॐ

oṃ
tat savitur vareṇyaṃ
bhargo devasya dhīmahi
dhiyo yo naḥ pracodayāt
oṃ

Oṃ. On That Adored Divinity of Savitur
We Meditate, Which is a Luminescent Divinity
May it Illumine, Guide, and Inspire our Intellect Oṃ.

The power of this Mantra is that its sounds crystallize to help humanity overcome the suffering that results from desire and attachment, and that its Japa helps part the veil of sensory illusion by guiding and illuminating our intellect, just like the Sun dispels the darkness at dawn.

Of the original Gayatri Mantra, the Gayatri Mantras of the Deva that we intone for the Chakras maintain the 24-syllable structure divided into three

16 A selection of Mantras and Bhajans (devotional songs) is given in Appendix I.

lines, as well as the ending of lines two (dhimahi) and three (prachodayat). They are:

Ganesha Gayatri for Muladhara Chakra

ॐ तत् गणेशाय विद्महे
वक्रतुण्डाय धीमहि
तन्नो दन्ति प्रचोदयात् ॐ ||

oṃ tat gaṇēśāya vidmahē
vakratuṇḍāya dhīmahi
tannō danti prachōdayāt oṃ

I am aware of that great energy manifesting as Lord Ganesha (Gana-Isha). That powerful energy is important in order to break through the inertia that faces any new project. This Lord of the Ganas (the netherworld forces) is depicted as an elephant-headed deity with a bent trunk and single tusk. I meditate upon this powerful force. May this force bless me in all my evolutionary endeavors.

Brahma Gayatri for Swadhishthana Chakra

ॐ वेदात्मनाय विद्महे
हिरण्यगर्भाय धीमहि
तन्नो ब्रह्म प्रचोदयात् ॐ ||

oṃ vēdātmanāya vidmahē
hiraṇyagarbhāya dhīmahi
tannō brahma prachōdayāt oṃ

I am aware of that great energy manifesting as the four headed (to represent the four directions) Lord Brahma. That energy is the force of creativity and is the source of all Vedas (Rig, Yajur, Atarva, and Sama). This energy is the golden womb of creation and can be called the bioplasm (Prana) from which the Universe originated. I meditate upon this powerful force. May this force bless me in all my creative evolutionary endeavors.

Vishnu Gayatri for Manipura Chakra

ॐ नारायणाय विद्महे
वासुदेवाय धीमहि
तन्नो विष्णु प्रचोदयात् ॐ ||

oṃ nārāyaṇāya vidmahē
vāsudēvāya dhīmahi
tannō viṣṇu pracōdayāt oṃ

I am aware of that great energy manifesting as Lord Narayanaya. That energy that is the Lord of Man (Nara) and is the force of conservation and continuity in this Universe. This Lord of the entire Universe (Vasu-Deva) is depicted as Lord Vishnu. I meditate upon this powerful force. May this force bless me in the maintenance of all my evolutionary endeavors.

Rudra Gayatri for Anahata Chakra

ॐ तन् महेशाय विदमहे
महादेवाय धीमहि
तन्नो रुद्रः प्रचोदयात् ॐ ||

oṃ tanmahēśāya vidamahē
mahādēvāya dhīmahi
tanno rudraḥ pracōdayāt oṃ

I am aware of that great energy manifesting as the Lord (maha-isha). I meditate upon this powerful force that is the Great force of Rudra (the fierce form of Shiva). This powerful energy is required to combat challenges in our spiritual evolution. Evolutionary Change is difficult and requires great raw force to deal with some of the obstacles. May this force of goodness bless me and empower me in all my evolutionary endeavors.

Shiva Gayatri for Vishuddha Chakra

ॐ तत्पुरुषाय विद्महे
वाक् विशुद्धाय धीमहि
तन्न शिवः प्रचोदयात् ॐ ||

oṃ tatpuruṣāya vidmahē
vāk viśuddhāya dhīmahi
tanna śivaḥ: pracōdayāt oṃ

I am aware of that great Universal Soul (Maharishi Patanjali refers to God as a special Purusha having no human failings such as the Kleshas or Karmas). I meditate upon this powerful force that gives great purity to our speech through the Vishuddha Chakra. This powerful energy manifests as Lord Shiva, the Lord of Goodness, change, or auspiciousness (change implies destruction of the past that the present can manifest, and some translators wrongly mention Shiva as the destroyer). May this force of change bless me and be auspicious in all my evolutionary endeavors.

Hamsa Gayatri for Ajna Chakra

ॐ हंस हंसाय विद्महे
परम हंसाय धीमहि
तन्नो हंस: प्रचोदयात् ॐ ||

oṃ haṃsa haṃsāya vidmahē
parama haṃsāya dhīmahi
tanno haṃsaḥ pracōdayāt oṃ

I am aware of the great discerning power in the Universe that is represented by the Great Swan (Parama Hamsa—the realized One). I meditate upon this powerful force of discernment, an aspect of Buddhi-intellect, centered in the Ajna Chakra. The Ham-Sa mantra is the Ajapa Mantra repeated 21,600 times a day (15x60x24) by all living beings unconsciously on the out- and in-breath respectively. The sound of SA is the inspiration of the Divine Self and HAM the exhalation of the individual self that occurs on every breath. We are born on an in-breath and die on an out-breath. May this discerning energy bless me and be with me in all my evolutionary endeavors.

Sukshma Gayatri for Sahasrara Chakra

ॐ व्योम वयोमाय विद्महे
सूक्ष्म सूक्ष्माय धीमहि
तन्नो सूक्ष्म: प्रचोदयात् ॐ ||

oṃ vyōma vayōmāya vidmahē
sūkṣma sūkṣamāya dhīmahi
tannō sūkṣmaḥ pracōdayāt oṃ

I am aware of that great Universal force that exists beyond the beyond (Vyom-Vyomaya) in space. I meditate upon this powerful force that is the subtlest of the subtle (Sukshma-Sukshmaya) forces. This force is represented by Sahasrara Chakra and pervades the entire cosmos. May this great subtle force bless me with an understanding of all the subtle concepts in all my evolutionary endeavors.

The six lower Pinda Chakras and the Sahasrara Chakra are linked to our individuality and therefore to specific qualities of our physical, energetic, emotional, and mental bodies. Below is a schematic introduction to each (Bhavanani 2002; Bhavanani 2008a):[17]

1. Muladhara Chakra (mūlādhāra cakra), the "Lotus of Root Support and Stability"[18]

Dhara Bija Mantra: Lang
Dala Bija Mantras (Four Petals and Flows of Energy): Vang, Śang, Ṣang, Sang
Gayatri Mantra: Ganesha Gayatri (gāṇeśa gāyatrī)
Mandala Shape: Prithvi Mandala (Yellow Square/Cube)
Jnanendriya: Ghrāṇa (Nose)
Karmendriya: Pada (Sense of Locomotion)
Tanmatra: Gandha (Smell)
Mahabhuta: Prithvi or Bhumi (bhūmi) (Earth and the Solid State)
Nervous Plexus: Sacral Plexus
Endocrine Gland: Gonads (Testes and Ovaries)
Physical Relation: Base of the Spine
Yoga: Hatha Yoga
Pranayama: Prithvi Mandala Pranayama

17 Between May 2022 and July 2022, Dr. Ananda created a YouTube playlist "Dr. AnandaJi on the Chakras" as part of his series *Scintillating Saturdays*. Each week's videos can be enjoyed on his YouTube channel: www.youtube.com/@YogacharyaDrAnandaBhavanani

18 For each Chakra's Sanskrit phoneme, refer to the image "Pinda Chakras, Bija, and Tattwas."

Asanas: Vajra Asana, Sukha Asana, Siddha Asana (siddha āsana), and Padma Asana (padma āsana)
Qualities: Stability, Integration, Solidarity, and Cohesiveness

At the lowest level of the six Pinda Chakras, we have the Muladhara Chakra, the grossest vibrational wheel where we start our journey back to the Source, going from the gross through the subtle into the causal. The journey starts where we are, on this earthly planet. Mula (mūla) means the root and Adhara (ādhāra) means support, so this can be translated as "the Root Support," which comes from a sense of stability of being "rooted" on the earth. Even though this is the slowest of the energy wheels, it is still moving at 20 times the speed of light. To fully understand the speed of light is difficult. The simplest way to do so is to think of infinity. In life, we need stability and a firm foundation, which helps us to be cohesive and integrated.

2. Swadhishthana Chakra (svādhiṣṭhāna cakra), the "Lotus of One's Own Abode"

Dhara Bija Mantra: Vang
Dala Bija Mantra (Six Petals and Flows of Energy):
Bang, Bahang, Mang, Yang, Ṛang, Lang
Gayatri Mantra: Brahma Gayatri (brāhma gāyatrī)
Mandala Shape: Apas Mandala (Silvery Crescent Moon)
Jnanendriya: Jihva (Tongue)
Karmendriya: Pani (Sense of Dexterity)
Tanmatra: Rasana (Taste)
Mahabhuta: Apas (Water and the Liquid State)
Nervous Plexus: Hypogastric Plexus
Endocrine Gland: Adrenal Glands
Physical Relation: Pelvic Region
Yoga: Jnana Yoga
Pranayama: Apas Mandala Pranayama
Asanas: Supta Vajra Asana (supta vajra āsana) and Matsya Asana (matsya āsana)
Qualities: Flexibility, Diplomacy, and Equanimity

The second Chakra is Swadhishthana. Swa refers to the self, the sense of individuality, and Adhishthana (adhiṣṭhāna) refers to being firm; therefore, the translation refers to "being established in one's self." Swa refers to self-analysis, and we find this prefix in the Niyama of Swadhyaya (svādhyāya), the study of the scriptures, because through the vicissitudes of characters in epical stories, such as Arjuna in the *Bhagavad Gita*, or Nichiketa in the *Katha Upanishad*, we can relate our small self to something greater and keep courage. Swadhyaya is also "the study of the self to understand and to follow one's Dharma," Swadharma (svadharma), which implies living in tune with one's highest potential. It is at this center that we secrete, on the physical-physiological level, adrenaline when we are not "at ease" with ourselves for an activation of the sympathetic nervous system. We want to learn how to be comfortable and at peace with ourselves. This is an essential teaching related to Swadhishthana Chakra. This is a center where we learn to be "at ease with the self" through self-appraisal and by learning to act rather than react.

3. Manipura Chakra (maṇipūra cakra), the "Gem City Lotus"

Dhara Bija Mantra: Ṛang
Dala Bija Mantra (Ten Petals and Flows of Energy):
Ḍang, Ḍahang, Ṇang, Tang, Tahang, Dang, Dahang, Nang, Pang, Pahang
Gayatri Mantra: Vishnu Gayatri (viṣṇu gāyatrī)
Mandala Shape: Tejas Mandala (Inverted Red Triangle)
Jnanendriya: Chakshu (Eyes)
Karmendriya: Payu (Sense of Excretion)
Tanmatra: Rupa (Sight)
Mahabhuta: Agni or Tejas (Fire and the Thermal State)
Nervous Plexus: Solar Plexus
Endocrine Gland: Pancreas
Physical Relation: Navel Region
Yoga: Pranayama
Pranayama: Tejas Mandala Pranayama
Asanas: Dharmika Asana (dharmika āsana)
Qualities: Power, Passion, and Motivation

The third Chakra is Manipura Chakra. Mani (maṇi) means "gems," and Pura (pūra) means "a city." Manipura refers to the amazing brightness of a city full of gems and jewels that are lighting the whole sky. This is the center where the universal energy comes into us through a "psychic umbilical cord." We are Solar beings and this is our Solar Center, our Nabhi. From here, the energy is sent to all other parts of the body. This is the energy that drives us, that gives us passion and motivation. We need energy and optimism to have brightness in our life and carry on our activities in tune with our Dharma. It is at this center that we secrete, on the physical-physiological level, endogenous serotonin, part of the feel-good hormones.

4. Anahata Chakra (anāhata cakra), the "Lotus of Unstruck Sound"

Dhara Bija Mantra: Yang
Dala Bija Mantra (12 Petals and Flows of Energy):
Kang, Kahang, Gang, Gahang, Ṅang, Cang, Cahang,
Jang, Jahang, Ñang, Ṭang, Ṭahang
Gayatri Mantra: Rudra Gayatri (rudra gāyatrī)
Mandala Shape: Vayu Mandala (Blue Hexagon of Interlaced Triangles)
Jnanendriya: Tvak (Skin)
Karmendriya: Upastha (Sense of Reproduction)
Tanmatra: Sparsha (Touch)
Mahabhuta: Vayu (Air and the Gaseous State)
Nervous Plexus: Cardiac Plexus
Endocrine Gland: Thymus
Physical Relation: Heart Region
Yoga: Karma Yoga
Pranayama: Vayu Mandala Pranayama
Asanas: Ardha Matsyendra Asana (ardha matsyendra āsana),
Brahmadanda Asana (brahmadaṇḍa āsana), Vakra Asana
(vakra āsana), and Gomukha Asana (gomukha āsana)
Qualities: Compassion, Empathy, and Unconditional Love

The next Chakra is Anahata Chakra. The name of Anahata Chakra refers to that "unstruck sound," Anahata Nada, that we discussed in previous chapters, a sound that doesn't have a cause, that doesn't have a point of origin, and, therefore, is an eternal sound. It refers to the universal vibration that has always existed and will always exist, Nada, also known as Anahata Nada. At the physiological level, in the heart, there is the Sinoatrial Node, a muscle made of "pacemaker cells" that create a spontaneous generation of impulse beyond the need for an impulse. There is a coupling of the cardiac function and the inhale and exhale of breathing. By focusing on Pranayama practices such as the Soham Mantra (Chapter 1) and Pranava Pranayama (Chapter 2) we expand our awareness on the vital relationship between heartbeat and breathing.

To be able to "tune in to" this "unstruck sound," we need to open our hearts. Swamiji teaches that the spirit of the Guru dwells within this Chakra. At this level of awareness, we learn how to be in tune with the universal vibration, to dance to the universal music so that we can move from being just an individual and can become part of a group, of society, of the world at large, and of the Universe. Relationship and companionship are key concepts in this center. We establish here a "heart-full" connection so that we can experience cosmic love and become true human beings.

5. Vishuddha Chakra (viśuddha cakra), the "Lotus of Great Purity"

Dhara Bija Mantra: Hang
Dala Bija Mantras (16 Petals and Flows of Energy):
Ang, Aang, Ing, Iing, Ung, Uung, Ṛing, Ṛiing, Ḷing,
Ḷiing, Eng, Aing, Ong, Aung, Aṁg, Ahang
Gayatri Mantra: Shiva Gayatri (śiva gāyatrī)
Mandala Shape: Akash Mandala (Magenta Oval)
Jnanendriya: Shotra (Ears)
Karmendriya: Vac (Sense of Communication)
Tanmatra: Shabda (Hearing)
Mahabhuta: Akash (Space-Ether-Sky and the Ethereal State)
Nervous Plexus: Pharyngeal Plexus
Endocrine Gland: Thyroid and Parathyroid Glands
Physical Relation: Throat Region
Yoga: Ashtanga Yoga/Raja Yoga
Pranayama: Akash Mandala Pranayama

Asanas: Sarvanga Asana (sarvāṅga āsana)
Qualities: Freedom, Transformation, Active Listening, and Vocalization

The next center is Vishuddha Chakra. Shuddha (śuddha) refers to purity and cleanliness, and Vi functions as a superlative, as in "great" and "absolute," on all levels of being. This is a center of great metaphysical as well as physical purity where discrimination and separation no longer occur. We step up through the ladder of consciousness: from the solid state of Muladhara, through the fluid state of Swadhishthana, the combustive state of Manipura, and the gaseous state of Anahata, we are now accessing the pure ethereal state of Vishuddha. This is the center of Akasha Tattva, a "space" where creation can manifest, and it is therefore psychically related to the mother's womb. Space is not "up there" but everywhere.

At the level of the nervous system, this center corresponds to the laryngeal plexus in the area of the neck. Here is the highest degree of freedom where hearing becomes listening and listening supports a healthy and empathic quality of communication. Our communication should be filled with gratitude, respect, love, and sharing. This is a very important development we all need. Rather than "what we can get," we choose to focus on "what we can give." This is "unblemished" communication for the sake of communication itself.

6. Ajna Chakra (ājñā cakra), the "Lotus of Intuition"

Dhara Bija Mantra: Ang
Dala Bija Mantras (Two Petals and Flows of Energy): Hang, Kṣang
Gayatri Mantra: Hamsa Gayatri (haṃsa gāyatrī)
Mandala Shape: Orange Circle
Element: Manas (Mind)
Nervous Plexus: Cavernous Plexus
Endocrine Gland: Pituitary Gland
Physical Relation: Between the Eyebrows
Yoga: Mudra Yoga
Pranayama: Manas Mandala Pranayama
Asanas: Padma Asana in Shirsha Asana (śīrṣa āsana)
Qualities: Relaxed Concentration

The next Chakra is Ajna, the sixth and last of the Pinda Chakras. Jna (jñā) refers to that knowledge that we gain in our day-to-day life, and a-, a negation, does not mean lack of knowledge but, rather, transcendence. We are withdrawing from daily knowledge and gaining wisdom from insight and intuition. When we move from Muladhara to Vishuddha, from earth to ether, we experience the densest element with the slowest speed of vibration all the way to the most refined element at the highest speed of vibration. In between these two polar opposites, we move clockwise around the cerebrospinal axis, the Sushumna Nadi, from earth to water, from water to fire, from fire to air, from air to ether. When we reach Ajna Chakra, at the middle of our eyebrows, we reach a super-element, the mind, Manas, and the movement of the energy is no longer spiraling but oscillating between its two petals, left to right. The two petals correspond to the two hemispheres of the brain, and the quantitative and qualitative aspects of our lives.

At Ajna Chakra there is a quantum leap from instinctive behavior that is reactive and reflexive to intuitive behavior that is responsive and reflective. This Chakra also has a Bindu, a subtle pinpoint passage between the Manomaya Kosha and the Anandamaya Kosha, called the Ajna Bindu, which, at the physical level, correlates to the thalamo-pituitary axis, that enables all the psycho-neuro-physiology to function. Mind, in Tantric Yoga teachings, is the sixth element, a higher level of perception. All the senses—whether smell, taste, hearing, sight, or touch—only operate when the mind is working. If the mind is shut off, the sensory apparatus falls flat. Finally, we are able to access the wisdom within ourselves, our power of discernment, Viveka (viveka). Swamiji often said, "every knowledge, everything in the Universe, is already within you." This is the real meaning of education, from the Latin verb "educare," which means "to bring forth knowledge that is already inside the student."

7. Sahasrara Chakra (sahasrāra cakra), the "Thousand-Petalled Lotus"

Dhara Bija Mantra: AUM

Dala Bija Mantra (One Thousand Petals and Flows of Energy): All of the 50 Sanskrit Phonemes repeated 20 times as a representative number. By invoking the sounds of the lower Pinda Chakra Dala Bijas, we create the "after-tone" for the higher Anda Chakras

Gayatri Mantra: Sukshma Gayatri (sūkṣma gāyatrī)
Mandala Shape: A Lotus of a Thousand Petals
Element: Atman (Soul)
Nervous System: Forebrain
Endocrine Gland: Pineal Gland
Physical Relation: Top of the Head
Yoga: Mantra Yoga
Pranayama: Pranava Pranayama
Asanas: Yoga Mudra Asana (yoga mudrā āsana) and
Baddha Padma Asana (baddha padma āsana)

At the seventh level we find Sahasrara Chakra, which means the thousand-petalled lotus, from Sahasrara (sahasrāra), which means "a thousand." This is a poetic expression for the concept of an infinite number of petals and not exactly 1000. Sahasrara is sometimes represented as a petalled lotus covering the head, but Swamiji taught us to activate this Chakra by restoring its traditional depiction as a crown, reminiscent of the aura of Christian saints.

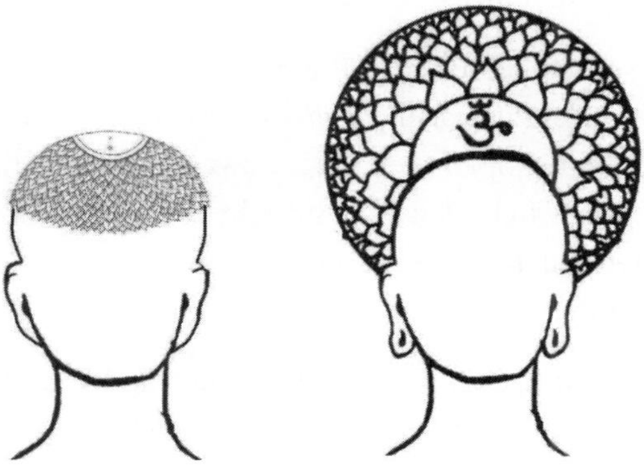

The Petals of Sahasrara

This number refers symbolically to the infinite capacity of our brain and the infinite connections that happen here at the neurological level. All our neurons are connected to each other—millions and billions and trillions!

Nada Yoga Practice

The following two practices were originally published in Lesson Thirteen of *Yoga: Step-by-Step* (Giri, 1976, A-49–50).

Shat Chakra Pranayama

On an in-coming breath, visualize the Pranic energy rising from the base of the spine up through six Chakras along the spine, and the descent of the Prana down through the same six Chakras on an out-going breath. Imagine that your body is a six-storied building and the Prana is rising and descending on an elevator lift. A held-in and a held-out breath can be added appropriately at the "back of the brow" center Ajna Chakra and at the base of the spine, Muladhara Chakra.

Chakra Meditation

1. Kneel in Vajra Asana, or take up any sitting posture in which you are absolutely certain that the spine is Yogically erect so that the energy can move upwards.

2. Do some deep Chakra Pranayama. As you come up through seven Chakras, starting from the base of the spine and through to beyond the top of the head, be aware of each of these centers, if only in the lightest way. In time, because of other practices, these centers will become conscious centers and fill with light, sound, and color.

3. When the breath is completely filled, and you are in Sahasrara Chakra beyond the top of the head, hold the breath in a Prana Kumbhaka, a held-in breath, for a lengthy period of time, then let out the breath and keep your concentration in that Thousand-Petalled Lotus Chakra.

4. Let the breath take on any form which it wishes and, simply, hold the idea that you are sitting in the midst of a beautiful Thousand-Petalled Pink Lotus. Hold that idea as long as you can, repeating the visualization over and over until a pleasing sensation of "being suspended" comes about.

This is a "sitting" meditation, and when taking up your Asana be sure to be facing North, other than just before the sunrise, when you can be facing East. Doing Shava Asana (śava āsana) just beforehand with deep conscious Pranayama can enhance this sitting meditation. The early forms of preliminary concentration and meditation are on and through the lower Chakras associated with the physical nervous system and the glandular bodies. There are a number of concentration and meditation techniques to do with the Mahakarana Chakras, the Great Causal Centers, which represent the Chakras Seven through Twelve.

Dhara Bija Mantra Japa Sadhana[19]

Practice 1: One Dhara Bija Mantra at a Time

1. Sit in a comfortable position, in a cross-legged Asana such as Sukha Asana or Padma Asana.
2. Align your spine and concentrate on your breath in a Sukha Pranayama.
3. Bring your hands in the Namaskara Mudra and invoke one Pranava AUM.
4. Invoke the Guru Gayatri Mantra and give thanks to the Gurus of the Parampara.[20]
5. Invoke one Gayatri Mantra for that Chakra, for example the Ganesha Gayatri Mantra for Muladhara Chakra, while focusing on the area inside and around the body corresponding to that Chakra.
6. Relax the hands and perform the Jnana Mudra (jñāna mudrā) with the hands on the inner thigh, at the knee, or simply rest your hands on your thighs.

19 Transcribed from the direct teachings of Yogacharya Dr. Ananda Balayogi Bhavanani by Yogacharini Dr. Sangeeta Laura Biagi from Dr. Ananda's Teachings during Module 3, Session 3, of the online Nada Yoga Immersion (March 3, 2022).

20 In Gitananda Yoga, the Guru Gayatri Mantra is invoked at the beginning of each session. You can find the Mantra in Appendix I.

7. Inhale and, as you exhale, while focusing on that Chakra, invoke the sound of that Chakra Dhara Bija Mantra, for example LANG for Muladhara. The first part of the Mantra, LA, is an expansion of the sound from the center of the body outwards. It is like the pebble dropping at the center of a quiet pond and from which waves ripple out in 360 degrees. When you are halfway through your exhale capacity, begin to "bring the sound back" from the outer environment back into the center of the body as you invoke the nasal-cerebral sound NG.

8. Perform nine rounds slowly, one breath per repetition.

9. Bring your hands in the Namaskara Mudra and intone one Pranava AUM.

10. Conclude the practice by invoking a Mantra for serenity and peace.[21]

Repeat this sequence for the other Chakras, always from Muladhara (first) to Sahasrara (seventh).

Practice 2: Combination Sequence of All Dhara Bija Mantras, Slow to Faster

1. Sit in a comfortable position, in a cross-legged Asana such as Sukha Asana or Padma Asana.

2. Align your spine and concentrate on your breath in a Sukha Pranayama.

3. Bring your hands in the Namaskara Mudra and invoke one Pranava AUM.

4. Invoke the Guru Gayatri Mantra and give thanks to the Gurus of the Parampara.

5. Invoke the seven Gayatri Mantras for the Divinities residing in the Chakras, in a sequence, from Muladhara to Sahasrara Chakra.

---

21 In Gitananda Yoga, the Lokha Samastha Mantra is invoked at the end of each session. You can find this Mantra in Appendix I.

6. Relax the hands and perform the Jnana Mudra with the hands on the inner thigh at the knee, or simply rest your hands on your thighs.

7. Invoke the Dhara Bija Mantras, always from Muladhara to Sahasrara Chakra—Lang, Vang, Rang, Yang, Hang, Aang, Om—in this sequence, one per breath.

8. Move the focus on each Chakra's corresponding area in and around the body.

9. The first part of the Mantras—La, Va, Ra, Ya, Ha, Aa, O—is an expansion of the sound from the center of the body outwards. It is like the pebble dropping at the center of a quiet pond and from which waves ripple out in 360 degrees. When you are halfway through your exhale capacity, begin to "bring the sound back" from the outer environment back into the center of the body as you invoke the nasal-cerebral sound NG.

10. Pick up the speed and repeat the Mantras one after the other, faster and faster.

11. When you have reached the fastest you can go, inhale and, *on the inhale*, make the sound of the Bija Mantras—Lang, Vang, Rang, Yang, Hang, Aang, Om—as if you were "gulping the sound up" while you feel and imagine you are bringing the breath all the way up to Trikuti Bindu, above the top of your head. Lower your chin down a bit in a gentle (not full) Jalandhara Bandha (jalandhara bandha), a "lock at the throat."

12. Hold the breath in (prāṇa kumbhaka).

13. Exhale and release the jugular knot, and on the out-breath, invoke the Pranava AUM while bringing your focus from Trikuti, at the top of the skull, down to the bottom of the spine and back to the top of the spine.

14. Keep your focus gently at the top of the skull to experience a mild version of Kevala Kumbhaka, a natural and comfortable suspension of the breath.

15. Bring your hands in the Namaskara Mudra and intone one Pranava AUM.
16. Conclude the practice by invoking a Mantra for serenity and peace.

Chapter 4

NADA YOGA CHIKITSA

"Healing with Sound"

Yoga, with its philosophies and practices, has assumed significance worldwide and so has Yoga Therapy, the English translation of the Sanskrit Yoga Chikitsa. The Government of India is currently promoting indigenous systems of health and healing including Yoga through the Ministry of Ayush. Yogamaharishi Dr. Swami Gitananda Giri, who was a medical doctor as well as a Yoga Guru, paved the road in bridging "Eastern and Western" medical approaches to health as an integrated system of body, emotions, mind, and spirit. Yoga Chikitsa he taught:

> is virtually as old as Yoga itself, indeed, the "return of mind that feels separated from the Universe in which it exists" represents the first integrated therapy. Yoga Chikitsa could be termed as "man's first attempt at unitive understanding of mind-emotions-physical distress and is the oldest holistic concept and therapy in the world." (Bhavanani, 2013b, p.29)

His son and successor, Yogacharya Dr. Ananda Balayogi Bhavanani, also a qualified medical doctor and esteemed Yoga Acharya, has been at the forefront of worldwide research projects in Yoga Therapy over the last two decades. With more than 300 scientific publications to his credit, Dr. Ananda has led the Centre for Yoga Therapy, Education and Research (CYTER) of Sri Balaji Vidyapeeth, promoting health in a holistic manner with a scientific research-based approach through its constituent Mahatma Gandhi Medical College and Research Institute (MGMCRI) in Pondicherry, India, since 2010. The innovative focus of CYTER has been on "salutogenesis," the concept of health promotion and disease prevention and management. This integrative approach bridges traditional and modern approaches to healthcare in the form of Traditional, Complementary, and Integrative Medicine (TCI) to serve the patient population in a more efficient, cost-effective, and patient-friendly manner.

In the fall of 2022, Dr. Ananda and his team inaugurated the Institute of Salutogenesis and Complementary Medicine (ISCM) at Sri Balaji Vidyapeeth, merging the CYTER, now upgraded as the School of Yoga Therapy (SoYT), with the School of Music Therapy (SoMT), that was previously functioning since 2010 as the Center for Music Therapy Education and Research (CMTER). In January 2023, Dr. Ananda and his illustrious team at ISCM successfully launched the 2nd International Health Research Convention 2023 and the International Conference on Role of Yoga and Music Therapies in Promoting Salutogenesis, which saw the participation of dozens of music and yoga therapy organizations and institutes, with hundreds of scholars, professors, teachers, and students from around the world.

The teachings of Yoga Chikitsa are so vast that one book would not be enough to cover this topic. The same can be said for Music Therapy and, in particular, the positive effect that music making, chanting, and singing have on human health. This chapter discusses some important concepts such as "health," "stress," "stress response," "stress management," and "relaxation" in light of traditional Yoga teachings and offers a sequence of four Nada Yoga practices (Sukha Pranayama, Nasarga Mukha Bhastrika, Shabda Pratyahara Kriya, and Pranava Pranayama) to help promote Yogic relaxation for health and well-being, supported by the results of current medical research at ISCM. We hope that this chapter will inspire Yoga practitioners, Yoga teachers, and Yoga and Music Therapists to incorporate some of these teachings in their own Sadhana and professional work.

Health is Spiritual

Health is an English word that derives from the Old English "hælþ," from which the verb "to heal" also derives, and that means "to be whole, to be well." Health implies a sense of unity with the self and the ease that derives from it. Vice versa, a lack of this cohesiveness may result in a feeling of disgregation and dis-ease. In 1948, right after the end of World War II, the World Health Organization (WHO) gave a definition of health in its Constitution as "a state of complete physical, mental and social well-being, not merely the absence of disease or infirmity" (WHO, 2023). This definition, in the context of "Western" medicine, marked a new understanding of health and well-being, not as a negation of pathology but as an affirmation of an interdependent system of experiences in the lives of individuals (physical and mental) and the role they play in society (social). This was a breakthrough in the West where allopathic medicine had mostly focused on symptoms of illnesses rather than on integrated well-being.

From the point of view of an "ageless" system of philosophy such as the Yoga Darshana, however, this definition is incomplete because it does not include spiritual well-being.[1] In the system of the Panchakosha,[2] for example, the physical body (annamayakośa) and the mental body (manomayakośa) are only two out of five "energy sheaths." One could make a correlation between the "social" body and the "energy" Pranic body (prāṇamayakośa) in the sense that we express and explore emotions and energy not only with ourselves but, perhaps more importantly, in relation to others. Even in this case, the two higher bodies of "intellect and wisdom" (vijñānamayakoṣa) and bliss (ānandamayakoṣa), which we could name, in a very simplified sense, the "spiritual bodies" or spiritual dimensions of a person's existence, need to be included in a wholesome understanding of "complete well-being."

In Lesson Ten of *Yoga: Step-by-Step*, Swami Gitananda writes:

> When the cosmic egg, Anandamaya Kosha, is perfectly centered by the lower bodies, then Samyam, or equilibrium, is said to exist. For the physical body it represents homeostasis, or organic equilibrium. It represents Sambhava, mental equipoise, for the mind with all the senses balanced and under control of the Buddhi, the higher, spiritual intellect. (Giri, 1976, p.A-37)

This alignment requires moment-by-moment awareness and a commitment to "be well." If not, Nara, "psychic dis-association," occurs:

> If the physical body is inharmonious with the higher bodies, accidents and physical illness are present. If the vital body is out of line, all sorts of

1 Spiritual comes from the Latin "spiritus," which means "breath" and also "inspiration" in a physical and metaphysical sense. "Spiritual" differs from "religious" because religion is an organized system of beliefs and practices, while spirituality is rooted in a personal relationship with the self and the Self, a greater intelligence or cosmic energy that may be named differently in different cultures.

2 See Chapter 3.

> emotional and psychic distortions are to be seen. Mental states occur when the lower mind body is out of line with its lower counterparts. If all three lower bodies are out of line with the higher mental body and the cosmic sheath, then untold tragedies occur. ... If the life of a Yogi is like "an arrow sent straight to its goal," then a state of total well being must be accomplished. Otherwise our efforts will go astray. (Giri, 1976, p.A-39)

Over the last few decades, the importance of spiritual well-being has been recognized by public health professionals, particularly the role it plays in the prevention and management of non-communicable diseases (NCD), such as cardiovascular diseases (heart attacks and stroke), cancers, chronic respiratory diseases (chronic obstructive pulmonary disease and asthma), and diabetes (Dhar *et al.*, 2013, p.3). Spiritual health relies on the capacity to be in the world while, at the same time, developing a sense of healthy detachment from the results of one's actions. Each person is both responsible for their choices and part of "something greater," a larger cosmic design, a higher intelligence that may be defined as God, Divinity, or the vibratory essence of a quantum field. According to Swami Kuvalayananda, founder of Kaivalyadhama, "positive health does not mean mere freedom from disease but is a jubilant and energetic way of living and feeling that is the peak state of well-being at all levels—physical, mental, emotional, social, and spiritual" (Bhavanani, 2017, p.44).

In Yoga, one of the terms for "health" is the Sanskrit term Swastha (svastha), a compound of Swa, "one's own, the self," and Astha (āsthā), "a place" and "to be established," which implies a sense of "being at ease with one's self" or, more poetically, "feeling at home with the self." Other terms in which we find the prefix "swa" are: the second of the Niyamas in Maharishi Patanjali's *Yoga Sutra*, Swadhyaya, referring to "study of the self," "study of spiritual teachings," and the second of three steps of Kriya Yoga (kriyā yoga); the name of the second Chakra, Swadhishthana Chakra, "the abode of one's self"; Swami (svāmī), the One who has Realized the Self through the self. Swa is a "sonic vibration" that embodies the relationship between the individual and the Universe, the microcosm of a person's finite life and the macrocosm of life's perennial energy. Dr. Ananda writes:

> According to tradition, yoga implies both the process as well as the attainment of a state of psychosomatic, harmony, and balance (samatvam yoga uchyate—*Bhagavad Gita*) and this restoration of physical, mental, emotional,

and spiritual balance may be the prime factor behind the changes seen across all short- and long-term studies. (Bhavanani, 2017, p.46)

In the teachings of Rishiculture Ashtanga Yoga, we learn that, for millennia, Yoga has provided an ancient system of "mind-body medicine" that has enabled individuals to attain and maintain Sukha Sthanam (sukha sthānaṃ), a dynamic sense of physical, mental, and spiritual well-being. Yoga, as a "way of life," is rooted in the Eternal Law of Dharma, according to which action is always met by a result and a consequence. "Regularity, rhythm, and repetition" are at the heart of a healthy lifestyle, as taught by Ammaji Yogacharini Meenakshi Devi Bhavanani. Regularity means living according to specific rules which, when repeated, create a rhythm in one's life. Life, health, and business coaches affirm the same: to build success, a disciplined routine is essential. Yet, in contemporary societies, many people are mistaking "individualistic freedom" for "lack of responsibility towards one's healthy rhythms." The advancements of technology and "modernization" allow us to work and live indoors with artificial sensorial stimuli and to drastically modify the natural times of rest and exertion, sleep and activity, eating and digesting with consequences that affect our well-being and our time and energy management skills.

Lifestyle modification is the keyword, and we must not forget that advice on diet and adoption of a healthy natural lifestyle are very important irrespective of the mode of therapy employed for the patient. The need of the modern age is to have an integrated approach towards all forms of therapy from Yoga Therapy and Music Therapy to allopathy, ayurveda, Siddha, homeopathy, and naturopathy. Physiotherapy, osteopathy, and chiropractic practices may be also used with the Yoga Chikitsa as required. A judicious blend is required, with a personalized and mindful approach to each individual.

"You Don't Have a Problem, You Are the Problem!": Yoga Bhavana

This is a very important teaching of Swami Gitananda. Life presents us with challenges. Some people experience extremely traumatic events and some don't, but overall, every human being is engaged in a "life and death" journey. Every moment could be our last and no one can predict the future. Each person's Dharma, the Swadharma, is regulated by the specificity of our cycle of birth/death/reincarnation and the fruits of our past actions (karma). The family, culture, time, and location of our current birth plays a great role in the formation of our personality. Swamiji wrote:

> The Law of Karma does not allow for such a thing as an accident. "Accidents are people looking for a place to happen" is one of my own pet expressions. Everything that happens in this Universe, happens under Divine Law. The Cosmos is orderly. Only human beings seem to be disorderly and chaotic. (Giri, 1976, p.73)

The three sources of Karma, in Swamiji's words (Giri, 1976, p.73), are as follows:

- Adhyatmika (ādhyātmika, pertaining to the Atma , ātmā, the "self"): Karma which is from the self and that arises within one's own actions, including "thoughts, daydreams, dreams at night, as well as acts of commission and those arising out of omission" (Giri, 1976, p.73). This source of Karma also includes actions from previous incarnations or early stages of this lifetime, such as childhood.
- Adhibhautika (ādhibhautika, pertaining to the Bhuta, bhūta, physical reality): Karma caused by "outside agencies" (Giri, 1976, p.73) in Nature, such as animals, weather, and natural catastrophes.
- Adhidaivika (ādhidaivika, pertaining to the deva, celestial planes and beings): Karma caused by Divine calamities. "The Devatas, Devis and Devas, are taken to be celestial gods and goddesses in Hinduism, but in actual fact, they are powerful psychic forces ruling the human mind and nervous system as well as the major glands of the body" (Giri, 1976, p.73).

Within such complexity, it is clear that we have little control over the events that occur each day and that "we will have to make the best of our Karma," which is a Law of Cause and Effect whose intricacies escape our rational judgment. Karma, when we make an effort to understand it, gives us the strength and momentum to manifest our Dharma. The two are not separate and Yoga is the heart of their union. If we fight or ignore our Karma and Dharma by breaking their Law, "unhappiness, sickness, disease and death" (Giri, 1976, p.77) will manifest. Yet, we are not victims to fate. Each life lesson pushes us towards our evolutionary goals. If what makes us human is the power of choice, what makes us *humane* is the courage to choose the best attitude towards ourselves, others, and life. This is the Yoga attitude of Pratipaksha Bhavana (pratiprakṣa-bhāvana), the cultivation of a constructive and positive attitude in the face of negative circumstances, as exposed by Maharishi Patanjali in the *Yoga Sutra*:

> [II:33]
>
> वितर्कबाधने प्रतिपक्षभावनम् ॥ ३३ ॥
>
> vitarka-bādhane pratipakṣa-bhāvanam
>
> *Cultivate the opposite attitudes when faced with negative tendencies* (Bhavanani, 2011a, p.163).

We have the power to choose our attitude. Dr. Ananda wrote:

> One practical aid is to tell one's self "Stop!" as soon as these negative thoughts surface. Even if we are not able to adopt the opposite attitude towards these deviant thoughts, we can at least make a conscious self-effort to stop them. Prevention is always better than cure. ... Do not let negative thoughts come in the door of your heartful-mind and mindful-heart! Pluck them out just like you would the weeds from your garden. (Bhavanani, 2011a, pp.163–164)

Swamiji wrote:

> To control one's personal Karma requires almost total awareness... an awareness that most human beings lack and that many do not even want. For many it is easier to turn a "blind-eye" to actions of others so that no one will criticize wrong actions on their part. There is no chance of Karmic evolution in that attitude. Awake! Be Aware! Mature! Grow! (Giri, 1976, p.69)

Swami Gitananda's "call to action" requires qualities of character that are essential for spiritual success and for a wholesome feeling of well-being. Maharishi Patanjali lists four of these qualities in *Sutra* I:20:

> [I:20]
>
> श्रद्धावीर्यस्मृतिसमाधिप्रज्ञापूर्वक इतरेषाम् ॥ २० ॥
>
> śraddhā-vīrya-smṛti samādhi-prajñā-pūrvaka itareṣām
>
> *The state of samadhi is attained by others through faith, valor, memory and equilibrium of the highest wisdom* (Bhavanani, 2011a, p.62).

Shraddha (śraddhā) means faithful devotion, faith, trust. This is a very important quality to cultivate and maintain for a sense of spiritual health.

Virya (vīryā) means strength of body and mind, valor, and it is necessary because the Yoga path is not always easy, and one needs strength to succeed. Smriti (smṛti) is the ability to remember and learn from previous experiences, another important quality that prevents us from making bad choices. Samadhi Prajna (samādhiprājña) refers to the highest wisdom rising from the state of Samadhi, a wisdom that can guide us in our evolutionary endeavors.

"Stress-Response-Ability"

Yoga Bhavana is an attitude that requires a sense of "response-ability" that is a keystone in the teachings of this Parampara. Each one of us must be "able to respond" to any circumstance with awareness, courage, and trust. One of the greatest gifts of Yogic Bhavana is that it teaches us how to become aware of, manage, and respond to stress. The term stress comes from the Latin "strictus," which means "tight." A simple yet comprehensive definition of stress, whose synonyms are tension and pressure, is offered by Dr. Ananda as "a huge expenditure of nerve energy" (Bhavanani, 2003, p.iii). Stress is not inherently bad. Good stress, eustress (from the Greek "eu," good), is essential for success, and it inspires us to accomplish goals and achieve optimal peak performance (optimal stress level). Bad stress, distress, is the experience of a continued level of high stress, which results in "burn-out." Eustress provides productive energy, increases focus, and feels exciting and manageable, while distress decreases performance and focus, and feels overwhelming and uncontrollable. In this sense, health is both a goal and a process in which we learn to manage the oscillations between distress and eustress and to move from focusing on pathogenesis (the development of dis-ease) to salutogenesis (the origin of health).

Salutogenesis is a neologism coined by Aaron Antonovsky (1923–1994), a professor of medical sociology who researched the relationship between health, stress, and coping (Antonovsky, 1979). It is a combination of the Latin "salus," which means health, and the Greek "genesis," which means the source, so it may be translated as "the origin of health." At the heart of salutogenesis is the "sense of coherence," which Antonovsky defined as:

> a global orientation that expresses the extent to which one has a pervasive, enduring though dynamic feeling of confidence that one's internal and external environments are predictable and that there is a high probability that things will work out as well as can be reasonably expected. (Antonovsky, 1979, p.123)

When we can look at our life and say "My world is understandable, manageable, and meaningful," we feel a sense of coherence. Coherence is a term that comes from Latin "co-haerere," "to stick together," and is a synonym of consistency. When we suffer because of pain, trauma, or fear, we experience a lack of the sense of coherence, a weakening sense of incoherence, a crumbling of certainties, and an upheaval of the regularity, rhythm, and repetition triad that makes our lives comfortable and comforting (from Latin "com-fortis," with strength). Incoherence results in a variety of lifestyle disorders.

Dr. Ananda writes:

> Yoga is the best lifestyle ever designed, it has potential in the prevention, management, and rehabilitation of prevalent lifestyle disorders. Yogic lifestyle, yogic diet, yogic attitudes, and various yogic practices help humans to strengthen themselves and develop positive health, thus enabling them to withstand stress better. This yogic "health insurance" is achieved by normalizing the perception of stress, optimizing the reaction to it, and by releasing the pent-up stress effectively through various yogic practices. (Bhavanani, 2017, p.42)

There is a useful correlation between these concepts as follows:

World is understandable	⇦⇨	Normalization of the perception of stress
Stress is manageable	⇦⇨	Optimization of one's reaction to stress
Challenges and overcoming them is meaningful	⇦⇨	Release of stress ("Do your best and leave the rest")

Thanks to Yoga Chikitsa, we can transform chronic stress (distress) into healthy stress (eustress). From lack of wellness, Yoga enables the abundance of wellness, which is spiritual bliss. As Swami Gitananda Giri reminded us, "Health and Happiness are our Birthright," and not a privilege of the few.

Our nervous system has two main divisions, the central nervous system (CNS), made of the spinal cord and the brain, and the peripheral nervous system (PNS), made of all the nerves that connect the brain and spinal cord to the rest of the body. A component of the PNS is the autonomic nervous system, which regulates involuntary physiologic processes including heart rate, blood pressure, respiration, digestion, and sexual arousal. It contains three anatomically distinct divisions: sympathetic, parasympathetic, and enteric. The sympathetic nervous system (SNS) and the parasympathetic nervous system (PSNS) contain both afferent and efferent fibers that provide sensory input and motor output, respectively, to the CNS.

The SNS controls our "fight, flight, or freeze" response to stressors. The physiology of the stress response (the way we respond to stress) follows this general flow:

Thoughts

⇩

Events ⇨ Perception of stress ⇦ Emotions

⇩

Stress

⇩

Hypothalamus

⇩

Pituitary gland
Release of the adrenocorticotropic hormone (ACTH)

⇩

Adrenal glands
Release of adrenaline, noradrenaline, and cortisol

⇩

Sympathetic discharge

⇩

Increased blood pressure
Increased basal metabolic rate
Increased blood sugar level
Increased muscle tone
Increased pupil dilation
Increased heart rate
Increased mental activity
Increased sweating
Decreased digestive processes

The PSNS controls our "rest and digest" processes by managing our body's response during times of relaxation. The signals of the PSNS travel through four cranial nerves (nerves that connect directly to the brain), one of which is the vagus nerve. Originating in the medulla oblongata of the brainstem, the vagus extends in the pharynx, larynx, neck, chest, and abdomen, innervating the voice box, lungs, heart, stomach, esophagus, liver, spleen, kidneys, intestines, and colon. These are vital internal organs that work "automatically" and whose dysfunctions alter our health in dramatic ways. Below the abdomen, through a neuronal connection with other nerves, the vagus also controls the anus and bladder functions. Vagal tone is the optimal physiological functioning of this nerve.

Homeostasis, the harmonious balance between SNS and PSNS activities, is the key to healthy living. In Yoga the process of alternating activity and rest is at the heart of many esoteric teachings, for example in the Spanda-Nishpanda (spanda-niḥspanda) principles of Tantra,[3] in the balancing of the active solar energy (ha) and the quiescent lunar energy (ṭha) in Hatha Yoga,[4] in the relationship between inhalation, exhalation, and breath retention in Pranayama, and in the coupling of Abhyasa and Vairagya, disciplined effort and detachment from results, in the *Yoga Sutra* of Maharishi Patanjali. We experience this process from birth until death thanks to our heartbeat. The heart is constantly in a pumping polarity between the active systole (Shpanda), during which it contracts and sends blood to the whole body, and the relaxation diastole (Nishpanda), where it supplies and nourishes itself. When the heart beats faster and faster, the time for diastole becomes less. The faster our heart goes, the less it supplies itself. The slower the heart beats, the more it is nourished.

Nada Yoga practices that involve expressed vocal sound are based on the regulation of the breathing cycle. Whenever we breathe in, our heart rate tends to be faster. Whenever we breathe out, our heart rate is slower. This

---

3 In very general terms, Spanda means vibration, expansion, generation, and Nishpanda means the related opposite of the withdrawal and reabsorption of that vibratory action.

4 Here is one of Swami Gitananda's teachings on these forces: "The term 'Hatha' is made up of two Sanskrit syllables 'Ha' and 'Tha'. The 'Ha' stands for solar forces in the body and specifically, positive Pranic forces flowing through the right hand side of the nervous system, while 'Tha' stands for lunar energy or more specifically, negative electromagnetic energy flowing through the left side of the nervous system. When the 'Ha forces' and the 'Tha forces' are balanced together as 'Hatha', perfect balance occurs (pronunciation 'Hat-ha not 'Ha-Tha')" (Giri, 1976, p.30).

is known as sinus arrhythmia in medical physiology. There is a theory that when we breathe in, the SNS is activated, and when we breathe out, the PSNS is more active. When people are under stress or tension, they tend to breathe in more rapidly. When we breathe in and out, there are pressure changes inside our chest. On an inhale, the chest cavity expands, the inner pressure is lower, and the blood from the abdominal area is pulled up because of the decrease in the pressure. When more blood is rushing to the chest, the SNS is alerting the heart to pump faster than usual. When we breathe out, on the other hand, there is more pressure in the chest cavity, blood is pushed out, and a relative decrease in the heart rate occurs. When we prolong our exhalations, we calm ourselves down.

When we invoke the sounds of Mantra, when we chant a Bhajan, a devotional song, our exhalation is longer than the inhalation, resulting in an activation of the PSNS and a related sense of ease and relaxation. In a pioneering study, published in the *British Medical Journal*, Professor Luciano Bernardi and colleagues from the University of Pavia, Italy, reported the effect of prayer and yoga mantras on autonomic cardiovascular rhythms (Bernardi *et al.*, 2001). They recorded breathing rates in 23 adults during normal talking, recitation of the Ave Maria prayer, yoga mantras, and controlled breathing. Breathing was more regular when the Ave Maria was repeated 50 times in Latin and when the mantra "om-mani-padme-om" was chanted. Both prayer and mantra caused striking, powerful, and synchronous increases in existing cardiovascular rhythms when recited six times a minute. This recitation slowed respiration and enhanced heart rate variability and baroreflex sensitivity, providing a feeling of calm and ease, and promoting physical as well as emotional, mental, and spiritual well-being. Choosing to stabilize the breath and invoking sounds to "entrain"[5] wandering thoughts results in a relaxation that is essential to salutogenesis.[6] Moreover, prolonged exhalation with vibration adds an extra benefit to our health, which is the

5 To learn more about sonic "entrainment" see Chapter 1.

6 The term "relaxation response" was coined by Dr. Herbert Benson, professor, cardiologist, and founder of Harvard's Mind/Body Medical Institute (Benson, 1975). Dr. Benson experimented and described the scientific benefits of relaxation as a treatment for a wide range of chronic stress-related disorders such as fibromyalgia, gastrointestinal ailments, insomnia, hypertension, and anxiety disorders. Many of Benson's exercises, drawn from Yoga, Buddhism, early Christianity, and Judaism and secularized for the purpose of his medical research in the United States, were rooted in meditative practices that involved breathing control and the sound repetitions.

production of endogenous nitric oxide that enables our sinuses to open and let air move through them. Similarly, thanks to humming sounds that are present in Mantras, blood vessels relax and dilate.

Over the last few decades, scientific research has confirmed what the Rishis of Sanatana Dharma and the Gurus of traditional lineages have taught all along: including sound in our Sadhana deepens perception, enhances focus and reduces distraction, awakens latent areas and develops neuroplasticity, balances hemispheric activity, helps develop associative understanding of interconnectivity, and enhances a sense of ease and well-being.[7]

The Gift of Yogic Relaxation

In the teachings of Rishiculture Ashtanga Yoga, great importance has always been given to Yoga Relaxation, which is at the center of most Raja Yoga practices. This form of relaxation is active and rooted in awareness, not a dull, inert form of "drooping away." Being and doing are one, integrated, united beyond disassociation. It is in this state of relaxation that healing, a wholesome process of rebalancing our physical, emotional, mental, and spiritual health, can occur. As long as we are in a "fight or flight" mode, we are unable to heal. Yogic relaxation is, without doubt, a gift to humanity and the greatest contribution to modern healthcare and wellness, because it impacts in a positive way the same psycho-neuro-immunology that was impacted negatively by stress. Yoga practices help us achieve an active relaxation whose effects are long lasting because they work on the symptoms (distress and tension) by uprooting their psychosomatic cause (ignorance and distorted perception).

Relaxation is not just a technique but a way in which we choose to live our lives. This is, of course, very difficult, particularly during times of grief, pain, and trauma, and Swamiji in his teachings kept reminding his students that the Yoga path requires tremendous courage and commitment. To support us on this path, this Parampara recommends healthy lifestyle choices that include: a healthy diet, appropriate hydration, regularity in eating and sleeping intervals, Hatha Yoga and Pranayama practices to stabilize one's metabolic activities, stress management through Yoga counseling, visualization, and

7 For a list of medical scientific studies on the benefits of Nada Yoga practices, see Appendix II.

contemplative practices to induce a sense of inner serenity, which include the invocation of prayers and Mantras. The effort to live a relaxed and healthy Yogic life is rewarded by meaningful results such as: improved quality of skin, vision, hair luster, sleep, memory, and digestion; improved immune system; restored circulation; improved emotional intelligence; mental clarity and focus; an increased zest for life.

Yoga Chikitsa: Adhi-Vyadhi

Yoga, as a spiritual mind-body therapy, understands the influence of the mind on the body as well as that of the body on the mind. The nature of the lower mind, the Chitta (citta), is to think in a rational way, to assess, organize, structure, and plan. This process is not inherently bad. However, when the lower mind is clouded by residual impressions from selected past experiences, we may "see" a threat when it is not there or anticipate that a stressor will represent itself even when that may not be the case. Depression and grief resulting from past memories and anxiety around future expectations affect our state of ease in the present moment. If this uneasiness becomes "the norm," dis-ease will ensue. It is therefore essential to learn how to manage one's perceptions, beginning with one's thoughts and, in particular, the process of identification with one's desires, problems, wealth, name, fame, spiritual achievements, or physical and mental illness.

The question of identification with inner and outer reality is at the heart of traditional Yoga teachings. One of Ammaji Yogacharini Meenakshi Devi Bhavanani's teachings is "witness the self without identification, justification, and condemnation." Teaching ourselves and others how to stop identifying with negative perceptions of our past, our life stories, and our dis-ease is a responsibility and privilege of Yoga teachers and therapists, and it can be translated to fit various professional and personal contexts. Dr. Sangeeta Laura Biagi, for example, integrated some of these Yoga-based concepts in her academic course "Healing Narratives" taught inside Cook County Jail in Chicago between 2017 and 2019. The Grammy-nominated short film *The Girl Inside*, produced by 1 Girl Revolution and Behold, documents the successful impact that this work had on the physical, emotional, mental, and spiritual health of the students inside the correctional facility (1 Girl Revolution, 2020).

Conscious and unconscious identification with our negative and destructive narratives, wrote Dr. Ananda in a study on the psychosomatic mechanisms of Yoga (Bhavanani, 2013a), when prolonged in time and intensified by repetition, may result in stress-related disorders that progress through four distinct phases:

1. Psychic Phase: This phase is marked by mild but persistent psychological and behavioural symptoms of stress like irritability, disturbed sleep and other minor symptoms. This phase can be correlated with Vijnanamaya Kosha and Manomaya Kosha. Yoga as a mind body therapy is very effective in this phase.

2. Psychosomatic Phase: If the stress continues there is an increase in symptoms, along with the appearance of generalized physiological symptoms such as occasional hypertension and tremors. This phase can be correlated with Manomaya Kosha and Pranamaya Kosha. Yoga as a mind body therapy is very effective in this phase.

3. Somatic Phase: This phase is marked by disturbed function of organs, particularly the target, or involved, organ. At this stage one begins to identify the diseased state. This phase can be correlated with Pranamaya Kosha and Annamaya Kosha. Yoga as a therapy is less effective in this phase and may need to be used in conjunction with other methods of treatment.

4. Organic Phase: This phase is marked by full manifestation of the diseased state, with pathological changes such as an ulcerated stomach or chronic hypertension, becoming manifest in their totality with their resultant complications. This phase can be correlated with the Annamaya Kosha as the disease has become fixed in the physical body. Yoga as a therapy has a palliative and "quality of life improving" effect in this phase. It also has positive emotional and psychological effects even in terminal and end of life situations. (Bhavanani, 2013a, pp.30–31)

It is therefore important to "catch" one's thought vibrations and eradicate them as they arise. The Samadhi Pada, the second of the four "chapter divisions" of the *Yoga Sutra* of Maharishi Patanjali, begins by defining Yoga as the cessation of the whirlpools (nirodhaḥ) of the subconscious and unconscious mind, the thought-vibrations of Chitta (cittavṛtti):

[I:2]

योगश्चित्तवृत्तिनिरोधः ॥२॥

yogaścittavṛttinirodhaḥ

Yoga is the cessation of the whirlpools of the subconscious mind (Bhavanani, 2011a, p.33).

Because of our identification with the Vritti (vṛtti sārūpyam) [I:4], we confuse the "seer" (us, when we experience our inner and outer reality) with our perception of the "seen" (the objects of desire). This is a necessary process of "mental purification" for the high realizations of Yoga, Union of the self with the Self.

In Sadhana Pada, the first 17 aphorisms encapsulate some very important teachings on the five human inborn psychological afflictions, the Pancha Kleshas, which manifest at various levels of severity and whose conscious management constitute, in what seems like a paradox, both a hindrance *and* the stepping stones of Yoga Sadhana towards the realization of Kaivalya. These afflictions are five tendencies that are so ingrained in us that we often mistake them for "normality":

[II:3]

अविद्यास्मितारागद्वेषाभिनिवेशाः क्लेशाः ॥३॥

avidyā-asmitā-rāga-dveṣa-abhiniveśaḥ kleśāḥ

These afflictions are ignorance, false identity, attraction, repulsion and survival instinct (Bhavanani, 2011a, p.112).

Ignorance (avidyā) is confusing the impermanent with the permanent, the unclean with the clean, the painful with pleasure, and the non-self with the true Self [II:5]. When this happens, we confuse the Truth with what is pleasant to "me," and a distorted sense of false identity (asmitā) begins to arise from a misidentification with the tool of perception [II:6]. It is the ego that develops a sense of attraction (rāga) to pleasure and repulsion (dveṣa) to pain and suffering [II.7–8], reinforcing our instinctual attachment to survival "at all costs" (abhiniveśaḥ). These afflictions are the "root" of our Karmic bondage manifesting through "perceived and un-perceived experiences of the present and future incarnations" [II:12] and, "as long as the root exists, fruitions manifest through class of birth, lifespan and experience of the sensory world" [II:13] with relative merits and demerits, "resulting in the fruits of the present and future" [II:14] (Bhavanani, 2011a, pp.125–128).

Dr. Ananda explains the relationship between mental agitations, Adji, and physical ailments, Vyadhi, by referencing the teachings of the *Laghu Yoga Vashishta* (laghu yoga vasiṣṭha):

> The Nirvana Prakarana of the Laghu Yoga Vashishta, one of the ancient Yoga Texts, describes in detail the origin and destruction of mental and bodily diseases. Sage Vashishta teaches Lord Rama that there are two major classifications of disease. Those that are caused by the mind are primary (adhija vyadhi, the psychosomatic, stress disorders) while those that afflict the body directly are secondary (anadhija vyadhi, infectious disease, accidents etc). The primary disease has two subdivisions. These are the Samanya (ordinary physical diseases) and the Sara (the essential disorder of rebirth that may only be destroyed by atma jnana or knowledge of the Divine Self). Samanya diseases are the ones that affect us physically and may be destroyed by the correction of the mind-body disharmony. It is in these psychosomatic disorders that the actual practical application of Yoga practices as a mode of therapy can be very useful. (Bhavanani, 2013a, p.29)

Kriya Yoga, the Yoga of action and purification, allows us to attenuate the impact of the Kleshas:

> [II:1]
>
> तपःस्वाध्यायेश्वरप्रणिधानानि क्रियायोगः ॥ १ ॥
>
> tapaḥ svādhyāy-eśvarapraṇidhānāni kriyā-yogaḥ
>
> *Kriya yoga consists of intensive self-discipline, introspective self-analysis and surrender to the Universal Will after doing one's best* (Bhavanani, 2011a, p.110).

Kriya Yoga is a refinement of perceptual vibrations from the grossest to the subtlest, from Kala (Tapah) to the Bindu (Swadhyaya) to the Nada (Ishvara Pranidhana).[8] Through the wisdom of Yoga, we move consciously from an attitude of identification with pain, suffering, and distress (duḥkha), and the resulting pathogenesis, to an attitude of sincere liberation from attachment, joy, gratitude, and relaxation, and the resulting salutogenesis.

8 Nada-Bindu-Kala; see Chapter 1.

The Yogic Concept of Origin of Disease

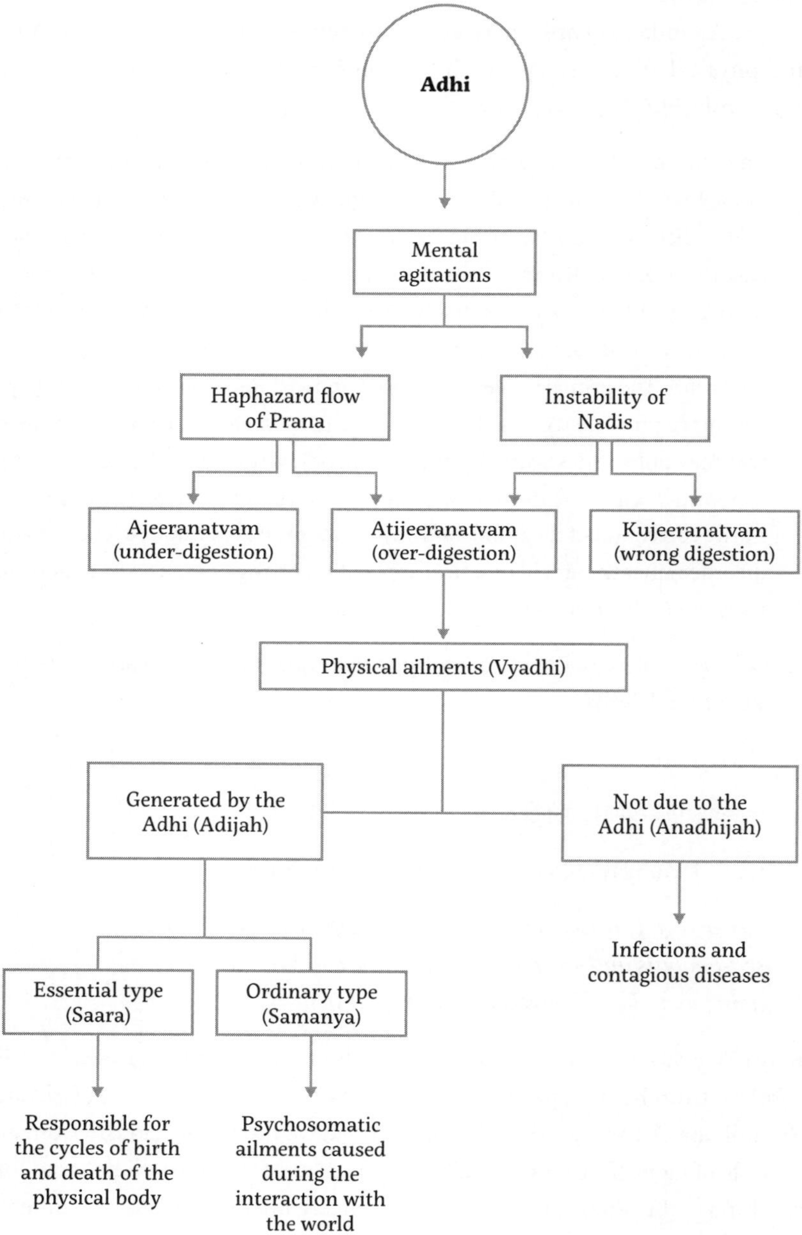

Adhi-Vyadhi

Nada Yoga: Practices for Health and Healing

In a conversation between Dr. Ananda and Dr. Sangeeta on Nada Yoga and the inclusion of its practices in Yoga Therapy, Dr. Ananda defined health as:

> the state of perfect oneness with the cosmic vibration. Illness is the result of dichotomy. When we are able to re-tune ourselves to the natural, universal vibrations, health occurs. We can think of health as a certain "state" of cosmic vibration. When we are "in tune" with that, and we are vibrating with it, we are truly happy and healthy. Every cell in our body vibrates in unison with that Divine vibration, and in that state, it is producing cosmic music, even if we cannot hear it. The music is always there but then we are not always attuned to it. When all our cells are vibrating as they should, producing the note that they should, we have a grand-symphony orchestra. Sometimes the cells go off tune and disharmony occurs. So all the nada yoga techniques are really aimed at enabling us to retune ourselves so that we can get back again into that balanced vibration. That is health. (Bhavanani and Biagi, 2013, p.10)

Listed below is a group of selected practices from the Rishiculture Ashtanga Yoga lineage that involve sound. Some of the beginning postures, which vary according to the practice, are:

- the standing posture of Samasthiti Asana (samasthiti āsana), the Equally Balanced Pose, with the chin up and open shoulders, the weight balanced equally on both feet, the palms facing the sun
- the sitting posture of Vajra Asana, the Thunderbolt Pose, where we put our weight on our heels and ankles, which are kept together. The palms are placed face down on the thighs
- the sitting posture of Sukha Asana, the Comfortable Pose, with the legs crossed at the ankles. The hands are clasped together in the Yoga Mudra, with the fingers of the right hand over the fingers of the left hand, or in the Jnana Mudra, with tip of the thumb and index finger gently touching, the other fingers extended, and the back of the hands on the inner thighs by the knees
- the sitting posture of Padma Asana, with the legs crossed so that the right foot is on the left thigh and the left foot is on the right thigh

- the face-prone position of Unmukha Asana (unmukha āsana), with the entire body in a straight line.

Bellows Breaths

Mukha Bhastrika (mukha bhastrikā)

Mukha Bhastrika, also called the Cleansing Breath, is a forceful expulsion of the breath to release carbon dioxide and other toxic waste matter from your bloodstream. The lips are puckered up in the Female Crow Beak Gesture, the Kaki Mudra (kākī mudrā). From Vajra Asana, inhale fully and blast out the breath in multiple whooshes (Bhastrikas) through upward movements of the diaphragm while slowly lowering the torso over the knees and bringing your forehead to the floor in front of your knees. Take one inhale and one full exhale. When you are ready to inhale again, lift your chin and inhale through the nostrils as you come back up to the Vajra Asana. Repeat three times. The third time, stay in the forward bend of Dharmika Asana, with the forehead on the floor and the nose between the knees. The arms are kept alongside the body with the hands catching hold of the heels. Concentrate on the point of the forehead that is touching the floor and visualize anything that you wish to remember well such as Mantras. This posture helps in the development of excellent memory power. Slowly, come back to the Vajra Asana on an in-breath. This Bellows Breath activates the solar plexus, thus strengthening the diaphragm and producing strength, vitality, and endurance.

Nasarga Mukha Bhastrika (nāsārga mukha bhastrikā)

Nasarga Mukha Bhastrika is a forceful expulsion of the breath through the mouth that can accompany different movements to relieve our pent-up stress. Take up a comfortable standing position and then start to shake your hands as vigorously as possible to help loosen up the accumulated tensions of your daily life. Visualize all the tensions that have accumulated in your wrist and elbow joints getting a good "shake up" by this action. When you have got the tensions loosened up, take in a deep breath through your nostrils and clench your fists as if catching hold of all your tensions and stress. Now, with a powerful blast through your mouth, "whoosh" away all your accumulated tensions and stress as forcibly as possible. Again, shake your hands as fast as possible. Breathe in and catch hold of the tension in your fists. Throw it all away with a blast. Make sure that you are using your diaphragm muscle vigorously while blasting out the breath. Perform this practice for three, six, or nine rounds as necessary and then relax in the standing position and enjoy the feeling of relief that sweeps through your body, emotions, and mind. This Bellows Breath activates the solar plexus, thus strengthening the diaphragm and producing strength, vitality, and endurance.

Kriyas

Hakara Kriya (hakāra kriyā)

This activating practice combines the use of movement with sound to give vent to pent-up emotional and mental stress by way of an effective release. It is also a good yoga warm-up. Stand in the Samasthiti Asana with your arms by your side. Breathe in and, at the same time, jump with your legs apart while clapping your hands over your head. Breathe out and make the explosive sound "HA" while jumping back to the standing position with the feet together and hands by the side. Do this six to nine times in a vigorous manner. Ha-kara is the production of the "HA" sound, which is related to the solar plexus. This plexus of nerves at the top of the abdomen is one of the centers where stress tends to accumulate. The strengthening of this area prevents the "butterflies in the stomach" feeling that occurs whenever we are stressed out. After completing the practice, relax back in the Samasthiti Asana and perform deep and controlled breathing for a few minutes. Enjoy the rejuvenating feeling as the energetic circulation of fresh blood rushes through your entire body.

Malla Kriya (malla kriyā)

This activity is loosely based upon the warm-ups done by Indian wrestlers to prepare them to face battle. It involves the use of the forceful Bhastrika breathing in synchrony with movement from the standing to the squatting position. Stand in the Samasthiti Asana and clasp your elbows in front of your chest with the right hand on the left arm and the left hand on the right arm. Take a deep breath in and then blast the breath out with a "whoosh" and, at the same time, come down to the squatting Utkat Asana (utkaṭ āsana). Breathe in and, at the same time, come back up to the standing position. Blast out the breath and go into the Utkat Asana. Breathe in and come back up to the standing position. Blast out and go into the Utkat Asana. Perform at least nine rounds of this practice. At the end of the Malla Kriya, relax in the Utkat Asana, the squatting posture that is valuable for the proper functioning of our abdominal and pelvic organs that make up our digestive and urinary systems. Your feet should be as flat to the ground as possible. Wind your arms tightly around your legs as if embracing yourself. Give yourself a good hug and feel the pressure that is generated in the abdominal region. All the organs are given a good massage and the whole digestive and urinary systems are invigorated. When ready, release the posture and come into any sitting position. Enjoy the renewed circulation of fresh blood in your abdomen and pelvis. Malla Kriya is valuable for those suffering with stress disorders such as diabetes mellitus, indigestion, irritable bowel syndrome, peptic ulceration, and impotency.

Pranayamas

Kukkriya Pranayama (kukkriyā prāṇāyāma)

Kukkriya Pranayama, the Dog Pant Breath, is an excellent cleanser and tones up the diaphragm and the abdominal organs that are in close proximity to the diaphragm. Sit in Vajra Asana with the weight of your body firmly on both heels. Place your palms on the ground in front with your wrists touching your knees and the fingers pointing forward. Open your mouth wide and push your tongue out as far as possible. Breathe in and out at a rapid rate with your tongue hanging out of your mouth. After ten or fifteen rounds, relax back into the Vajra Asana and feel the blood flow into your abdominal area. Repeat the whole practice three more times.

Bhramari Pranayama (bhramarī prāṇāyāma)

Bhramari is one of the Swara Pranayamas (svara prāṇāyāma) and helps tone up the nervous system, thus producing a state of extreme calmness and bliss. Bhramari is the female bee. The sound can be experienced on the exhalation at a low pitch, as the "female bee," Brahmari, and on the inhalation at a higher pitch, as the "male bee," Brahmara. It is performed sitting on the heels in Vajra Asana with your spine erect. This is a posture that grounds us and connects us to the earth. It is also performed with a special gesture, the Shanmukhi Mudra, the Mudra of "six perspectives," also named Yoni Mudra (yonī mudrā). In this Mudra we use the fingers of our hands to "close off" the sensorial inputs on our face. We make a conscious choice to use our hands, an extension of our heart, to focus on our spiritual life by connecting with ourselves. The thumbs are gently placed inside the external auditory canals; the index and middle fingers are placed over the closed eyelids; the ring fingers regulate the flow of air through the nostrils; the little fingers are placed over the closed lips. The five senses are therefore placed under the control of the conscious mind. With this practice, we move from the snare of the senses, Indriya-Jala (indriyajāla), to the victorious mastery over the senses, Indriya-Jaya (indriyajaya).

When we bring the hands on our face in this manner, we come into contact with the fifth cranial nerve, the trigeminal nerve. The base of the nerve is by the thumb location in the Mudra. The ophthalmic branch of the nerve travels to and above the eyes, the maxillary branch travels to the upper jaw, and the mandibular branch travels to the lower jaw area. The first two branches are responsible for sensory stimuli; the third branch is both sensory and motor, allowing the mandible to move in mastication and speech. This is an excellent example of a Pratyahara Mudra (pratyāhara mudrā) to withdraw our awareness back into the Inner Self. This mudra helps in uniting the energies of the nerves of the hands with the facial and trigeminal nerves of the face. Because we sit in Vajra Asana, we are also bringing under our awareness the action senses: the feet (locomotion), the hands (dexterity), and the organs of excretion (excretion), reproduction, and speech (communication).

Inhale deeply and, as you let out the breath very slowly, make a sound in the nasal passages like the high-pitched sound of a female bee. Perform nine rounds of this practice and then release your hands back to your thighs and enjoy a few minutes of deep contemplation while sitting in Vajra Asana. In Bhramari Pranayama, the relationship of the inhale and the exhale can be either 1:2 or 1:3 (i.e. breathe in for a count of 6 and then breathe out for a count of 12 or 18). The benefits of this Pranayama performed with the Yoni Mudra are many. Among the most important are: mental calm and clarity, serenity of emotions, reduced irritation and anger, lower blood pressure, improvement of vocal tone, improved self-esteem.

Pranava Pranayama

This practice, which was the focus of Chapter 3, is one-pointed concentration on the form and Nada of the sacred Pranava AUM, known as the Mantra of all Mantras. This can be done from any of the sitting postures but make sure that your back is erect. It is best to do this after performing a few rounds of conscious deep breathing so that the mind is in a calm state. It is an important part of the Rishiculture Ashtanga Yoga tradition as taught by Yogamaharishi Dr. Swami Gitananda Giri. In this practice, emphasis is placed on making the sounds "AAA," "UUU," and "MMM," first separately and then in combination. This is followed by the mental performance of the practice without the audible sound. A daily performance of three to nine rounds of the Pranava Pranayama helps to relax the body-emotion-mind complex and provides complete healing through the production of vibrations at all levels of our existence. This is the cornerstone of Yogic breath therapy. When the concentrative aspect of the practice is taken to its peak, a state of meditation or Pranava Dhyana (praṇava dhyāna) may ensue.

Mudras

Bhujangini Mudra (bhujaṅgīni mudrā)

To perform the "cobra gesture," take up the face-prone posture of Unmukha Asana. In this technique, the emphasis is on the breathing pattern and the production of a mighty hissing sound through the clenched teeth. Slowly bring your arms forward and keep your palms on the ground alongside your shoulders. Take in a deep breath. While making a mighty hissing sound, flare back into the Bhujanga Asana (bhujaṅga āsana). Slowly relax back onto the floor while breathing in and then again flare back with a mighty hiss. Repeat this Mudra at least three to six times at each session. This technique helps release the pent-up stress that accumulates in our systems from our daily life and provides great emotional and mental relief. It is an excellent stressbuster and is a must for all in this day and age. After completing the practice, come back down to the face-prone pose. Place your arms alongside your body and turn your head to the side. Relax for a few minutes and let the benefit of this Mudra seep into each and every cell of your body.

Brahma Mudra

This practice reminds us of the four heads of Lord Brahma, hence its name. It is a gesture of the head and neck that is excellent for cervical spinal problems. Sit up in Vajra Asana with your spine as aligned as possible. Rest your hands on your lap while performing the Yoga Mudra. Close your eyes and concentrate on this valuable practice that combines the use of physical movement synchronized with deep breathing and the use of the Nada vibrational sounds of the Bija "AAA," "UUU," "EEE," and "MMM." Breathe in and turn the head to the right side. Breathe out while bringing the head back to the central position and making the sound "AAA." Then breathe in and turn the head to the left side. Breathe out while bringing the head back to the central position and making the sound "UUU." Now breathe in and lift your chin as if to look at the ceiling. Elongate the neck without pinching the cervical area. Breathe out while bringing the head back to the central position and making the sound "EEE." Finally, breathe in and lower the head so that the chin touches the chest. Breathe out while bringing the head back to the central position and making the sound "MMM." Perform this practice a minimum of three times and a maximum of nine times at each sitting. Brahma Mudra is an excellent practice to prevent as well as relieve disorders of the head, neck, and upper shoulder areas. It is important to concentrate on the area to be relieved, repaired, or rejuvenated while sounding the Bija Mantras.

We conclude our practices with a relaxation in Shava Asana, the Corpse Pose, an energizing posture in which the body, emotions, and mind are united in the process of conscious relaxation. Fifteen minutes of Shava Asana properly performed is equal in relaxation to more than one hour of refreshing sleep:

1. Lie supine on a flat surface with the head preferably to the north or east, putting the body in alignment with the earth's magnetic field.

2. Make sure that the head and the feet are aligned and that the hands are relaxed by the sides of the thighs with the palms facing upwards.

3. Keep the legs and feet together with the heels touching lightly and then let the forefeet fall away into a "V" shape.

4. Witness the movement of the breath. Let your awareness settle

in the abdomen. Feel the cool air flow into the nostrils and the warm air flow out of the nostrils.

5. Let your awareness settle at the tip of the nose.

6. Regulate the breath on equal counts (4x4 or 6x6 or higher counts) and repeat one cycle nine times.

7. Enjoy the relaxed breathing for 10–15 minutes.

8. When you are ready to come back to action, slowly turn onto your left flank with your right flank dominant, and rest in a fetal position.

9. Turn onto the face-prone position of Unmukha Asana and perform the Makara Asana (makara āsana), the Crocodile Posture, by spreading your legs apart with the heels facing each other and toes facing outwards. Bring the left hand in front of the face with the palm touching the floor and keep the right hand over it. Place the chin or forehead on the back of the right hand and relax.

10. Bring the palms of the hands by the sides of the shoulders and perform the Bhujanga Asana, the Cobra Posture. Slowly lift the head and then raise the torso until the arms are straight, but do not lift the navel off the floor.

11. Lower the head and torso and lift the buttocks to transition into Chatushpada Asana (catuṣpāda āsana), the Four Footed Pose, with the palm of the hands and knees on the floor and back parallel to the floor. Inhale and exhale deeply a few times and then come back to the sitting Vajra Asana.

Mantras

In Chapters 2 and 3, we discussed the power that Mantras contain and express. When we invoke and evoke a Mantra with devotion and dedication: we connect spiritually with subtle psychic energies; the elevated sounds further focus and calm our mind; the rhythms of our breathing stabilize our emotions; we relax our bodies as we contain the animalistic urge to move about and, instead, sit up in a noble posture. Through Mantra Sadhana, we consciously remove the blocks that prevent us from connecting with ourselves, others, and greater forces. Mantra may be invoked by oneself and in a group, in a loud recitation or a whisper. A very powerful form of Mantra is the Manasika Japa (mānasika japa) or the silent repetition of a Mantra.

In the book *Saraswati's Pearls* (Bhavanani and Biagi, 2013), Dr. Ananda shares the effect that the repetition of the Om Namah Shivaya Mantra (oṃ namaḥ śivāya mantra) had on one of his patients:

> This makes me think of a patient who first came to me about nine years ago. He used to drink and smoke a lot. When he came to me, his heart vessels were almost completely blocked. He was a businessman and did not, in his perception, have time to practice. So we worked on a few small things. I asked him which Hindu God he preferred, and he told me Lord Shiva. So I told him to sit everyday and chant the mantra "Om Nama Shivaya" together with the practice of pranava pranayama, chandra nadi pranayama and some basic jathis and relaxation. After three years, he came back. He had gone to the cardiologist in Chennai and did all the scans for a check up. They found that all the blocks were still there, but the arteries had branched out and created collaterals around his heart, which was now getting all the blood it needed. We asked him what he had been doing and he said that daily in the morning and at night, he did 108 Om Namah Shivaya chanting. What happened is that to emit the sound of the mantra, his in breath was definitely shorter than his out breath, creating a ratio of at least 1:2 if not more. Therefore, his heart rate lowered, facilitating a larger supply for the heart to nourish itself while also stimulating the creation of the collaterals. (pp.15–16)

In the lineage of Swami Gitananda Giri, Mantras are invoked three times, nine times, or in multiples of nine. A Japa Mala (japa mālā) is a string with Rudraksha seeds (also referred to as beads), indigenous to India and of different colors, shapes, "faces" (segments), and sizes, each one containing a different energy, value, and symbolism (Giri, 2022). Traditionally, Malas have 108 beads, or half of that, 54, and are held with the right hand. Each bead corresponds to one Mantra recitation. Mantras are known by their name and by the number of their sacred syllables. For example, the Mantra for Lord Shiva may be referred to as the Om Namah Shivaya Mantra or as the Panchakshara Mantra, the Mantra with five (pañca) letters (akṣara), i.e. Na-Mah-Shi-Va-Ya.

Regarding the pronunciation of Mantras, particularly for those who did not grow up speaking Sanskrit or Tamil, both Swami Gitananda and Dr. Ananda have always been very clear regarding this point: the intention with which the Mantra is chanted, the Sankalpa, is as important as the correct pronunciation. Mantras are accessible to every sincere "seeker." The key is to be "worthy" of intoning a Mantra, and the way we become worthy is through dedicated self-effort: the effort to learn to pronounce the Mantra in the best way we can and not in a perfect way; the effort to understand the context of the Mantra together with its pronunciation; the effort to cultivate the best attitude and intention, the Sankalpa. What is our intention when invoking and evoking a Mantra? Is it to be the best version of ourselves? To make this world a better place? To be a comfort and support to others? Then, our Mantra will be powerful. If our intention is based in greed or jealousy, then no matter how great our pronunciation is, the Mantra's power will not be activated properly.

Appendix I contains a selection of Mantras that are invoked at Ananda Ashram, ICYER, and at Sri Kambaliswami Madam during the Pujas, ritual ceremonies held every Sunday, and on special occasions to celebrate the Gurus of the Parampara.

Bhajans

Bhajans are devotional songs, generally performed by groups of devotees in a "call and response" style, that celebrate the beauty, power, grace, and strength of the Hindu Devas (deva), gods and goddesses. When Bhajans are sung in special gatherings in temples or during special ceremonies, their power is to uplift the community through a choral experience—everyone is invited to sing and to lead, regardless of their training or experience as a singer. Dr. Ananda, during one of our online Nada Yoga classes, defined the experience of singing Bhajans as "emotional cathartic group therapy." In Bhajans the speed of repetition increases progressively, and so does the Bhava (bhāva), the feelings and sentiments (devotion, praise, love, adoration, gratitude) channeled through them. When Mantras become Bhajans, as in the example of "Om Namah Shivaya," Mantra Yoga and Bhakti Yoga[9] (bhakti yoga) merge.

9 The path of Yoga through devotion.

Karnatic Music and Yoga Sadhana

Music has been an instrument for health and healing since antiquity all around the world. Each culture has its music, and music changes cultures. Karnatic music (karṇāṭaka saṅgītam) is a style of devotional classical music that flourished in Southern India and retains a lot of the pure Indian cultural ethos and the Bhakti Bhava (bhakti bhava), the attitude of loving devotion. The performance of Indian classical music, vocal and instrumental, has been a very effective therapeutic tool in both Yoga Therapy and Music Therapy and its research is at the heart of the School of Music Therapy at the Institute of Salutogenesis and Complementary Medicine at Sri Balaji Vidyapeeth in Pondicherry directed by Dr. Ananda.

The seven notes, the Sapta Swaras (sapta svarāḥ), originate in the *Vedas* and are therefore timeless and not "written" by humans. Just like "seed mantras," they contain and evoke a specific energy and associations. The Swaras are Sa (ṣaḍjam, which means "giving birth to the next six notes"), Ri (ṛṣabhaḥ, "morality"), Ga (gāndhāraḥ, "fragrant"), Ma (madhyamaḥ, "the middle one"), Pa (pañcamaḥ, "the fifth"), Da (dhaivataḥ, "of the Devas"), and Ni (niṣādaḥ, "to sit/lie down"). Each Swara corresponds to a Western note, an animal, a color, a divinity, and an "emotional flavor and essence" (rasa).[10] Purandara Dasa (c.1470 CE–c.1565 CE) is known as the "grandfather of Karnatic music" (pitāmaha) and his stylistic choices codified Karnatic music as we still learn and enjoy it today. Three other composers, who are regarded as the "Trinity of Karnatic music," are Tyagaraja (1767–1847), Muthuswami Dikshitar (1776–1827), and Syama Sastri (1762–1827) who composed songs, Kritis, in Sanskrit, Telugu, and Kannada languages.

In Karnatic music, the two essential elements are Shruti, or tone, and Laya, rhythm. These are the two good parents of good music: Shruti is Mata (mātā), the mother, and Laya is Pita (pita), the father. If one of the two is missing, the music will be lacking. In Yoga, as we discussed previously, Shruti is also the quality of Vedic teachings, which are passed down orally, literally "through the tone." Each person's Shruti, or basic pitch, is different. The Shruti is the reference note, and it is "the mother" because

10 The Rasa theory was codified by Sage Bharata Muni in the Sanskrit *Natya Shastra* (nāṭya śāstra), a codification of rules for classical Indian theater, music, and dance. The nine Rasas are: Śṛṅgāraḥ, love and romantic affection; Hāsyam, laughter; Raudram, fury; Kāruṇyam, compassion; Bībhatsam, disgust; Bhayānakam, terror; Vīra, heroism; Adbhutam, wonder; Śāntam, calm and contentment.

it is through the maternal principle that everything manifests. Once we have the reference point, we move with the "father," the rhythm, the tempo, the Laya. Laya is the quality of space between the points. Music lies in the space between the notes, and rhythm lies in the space between beats. This musical system fosters relationship building in the present moment, as it is a constant dynamic interaction.

Swami Gitananda and Yoga Puduvai Shakti Meenakshi Devi Bhavanani, Ammaji, have, as per tradition, included the study and practice of the classical arts of India, particularly Karnatic music and Bharatanatyam dance in Yoga Sadhana. At Ananda Ashram, Karnatic music is an integral part of Yoga Sadhana and is taught by Yogacharini Devasena Bhavanani, Dr. Ananda's wife. The notes are revered as sacred and taught slowly, one by one, in a series of scales that develop focus, mental clarity, breath awareness, and sensorial expansion. As Ammaji teaches, music and dance are an emotional outlet, which may not be there in Yoga. It is important to express ourselves but within a disciplined structure. When learning Karnatic music, it is necessary to develop the correct posture (asana), to master breathing (pranayama), and to focus the mind for extended periods of time (dharana). The notes are learned one at a time, with respect and devotion. When we are able to be at ease with these fundamental steps, we may open up to the grace of experiencing bliss.

A Gem of Nada Yoga Chikitsa: Relaxation[11]

During Module 5 of the six-month online training in Gitananda Nada Yoga (2022), Yogacharya Dr. Ananda Balayogi Bhavanani shared Swami Gitananda's "Four Levels of Relaxation" (Giri, 1976, pp.113–114), a step-by-step method to become aware of stressors, release them, and open up to a higher Self. These teachings inspired Dr. Sangeeta to create a sequence of Nada Yoga practices that progressively instill deeper relaxation through intentional listening and vocal sounds. The practices are the ones shared earlier in the book: Sukha Pranayama, Soham Mantra, Nasarga Mukha Bhastrika, Shabda Pratyahara Kriya, and Pranava Pranayama. Swami Gitananda writes:

---

11 An early version of this section was originally published in *Yoga Life International Monthly Journal*, *53*, 8, 7–11, in August 2022, with the title "Swami Gitananda Four Fold Relaxation: Nada Yoga Practices."

Deep relaxation and Yoga are synonymous when we reach the inner phases of Yoga. For at this stage relaxation is not only body relaxation, but also a state where the physical body, emotions and mind are all brought up into a high state of conscious relaxation. … The Yoga system views the need for relaxation and its solution in four ways:

1. LETTING DOWN: This letting down is to deal with one's barriers to the needed advice and help, to let down one's prejudices and preconceived ideas and notions about people, things and ideas, to let down all of the false notions and materialistic idolatry that we have built up in modern living and in particular, to let down from the "God of Tension" which is virtually deified in "so-called" civilized society. To break away from the superstitions of our social and religious beliefs is not easy to do. These beliefs may be needed to support a healthy psyche. Therefore, it is necessary that you find out the truth, stripped of all false belief, about your own nature and the nature of the Supreme. Leave off all fears and anxieties and gain a positive attitude towards yourself and others. Cultivate the desire for right action when action is called for.

2. GIVING UP: One has to want to give up the stresses and strains that beset them. This does not mean a surrender or a defeat, as popularly suggested by the English term "to give up." This giving up is to throw off any weaknesses which tend to build up to tension and to give off or let off those foolish tensions that oftentimes turn us into a smoking volcano. Giving up here is a positive process.

3. GIVING IN: To give in, in the Yoga concept of relaxation, is to "give in" to the dictates of the inner mind, the Higher Consciousness. Again, this is a positive process and is not the giving in of surrender. There is no negation or abdication of positive actions and ideas. One has to take up an Inner Life study to understand what it really means in words to give in to the Inner Self. In the beginning, it is an intellectual process, highly exciting and satisfying, but it must move beyond the intellectual, ecstatic state to even a more positive, a more transcendental state.

4. GIVING OVER: The giving over of the control of the Higher Mind to the Higher Self is the highest and last stage of Four-Fold Relaxation.

> This is where the highest attainments of relaxation are achieved, where one can merge into beautiful super-conscious higher states of which you are aware, but no words can describe. Giving over represents the peak of fulfillment.

Four-Fold Relaxation peels off layers of stress, one by one, and allows us to relax and experience freedom from fear, anxiety, and worry. Becoming aware of the grossest vibrations of a distracted mind, we let go of emotional hang-ups, refine our Inner Mind, and ultimately, surrender to the intelligent laws that sustain the Cosmos as we know it. Relaxing at deeper and deeper levels requires a willingness and capacity to cleanse, purify, and quieten our Inner Self. Swamiji's clarity of exposition does not imply that the process of Four-Fold Relaxation is simple; on the contrary, most of us are barely aware of our negative thoughts and of destructive belief patterns emerging from unprocessed trauma. Even when we become aware, it takes conviction, faith, strength, and an undisturbed attention not to get sidetracked and distracted, and to decide to let go of our weaknesses.

Gitananda Nada Yoga practices give us accessible and practical tools to access these layers.

Letting Down: Sukha Pranayama—Soham Mantra

Preconceived ideas may come up as inner voices, thoughts, or beliefs. These have a noticeable effect in our bodies, so the first step in this Four-Fold Relaxation is to regulate the breath through Sukha Pranayama.

Sukha Pranayama

Breathe in and out through your nostrils, making your breath deep and even. Perform nine rounds of breathing in and out to a count of either 4x4 or 6x6, and begin to calm down and focus your mind. Observe any negative thoughts or habitual patterns of thinking that you are ready to dismantle and outgrow. Focus on them, rather than pushing them away. Remember that these thoughts—beliefs, false assumptions, negative voices—are part of what Maharishi Patanjali calls the Citta Vritti (*Yoga Sutra* I:2), "the fluctuations of the lower mind" (cittavṛtti). They can be heard, felt, or visualized. "Catch them" under the control of your mind and bring them to your awareness. Keep them there. They will resist.

Corral them, gently, as you would do a wild animal. Continue to breathe regularly, deeply, and with ease.

Giving Up: Nasarga Mukha Bhastrika

Giving up our habitual reaction to stress is not as easy as it may seem. When we are used to something, we become "used by it" and we may forget that living in a state of stress is not "normal." Thanks to the "whooshing sounds" and the movement of this practice, we shake off habits as well as stress. The whooshing sound, shaking, and gesture of "giving up" the worry and stress create a potent combination of breath, movement, and sound that is a special quality of the teachings of Rishiculture Ashtanga Yoga.

Nasarga Mukha Bhastrika

Begin with a Jathi (warm-up/de-stress practice) by shaking your right and left feet and legs, your buttocks and hips, your shoulders, arms, and hands, and your head, and then shake the entire body all at once. Have fun with the shaking, and be mindful of both pushing your comfort level and listening to your body. Then imagine that you are scooping up into your closed fist all the negative energies that weigh you down. Then, with a big inhalation through the nose (Nasa), "whoosh" them out with a sound through your mouth (Mukha): "Whooshh!" Please gesture this Kriya with feeling (Bhava), as if you are gathering up the thoughts and stress and casting them away. Do not "throw" these negativities at someone! Send them to the sky, the horizon, an open window, or the trees. Practice a total of three times or in multiples of three.

Giving In: Shabda Pratyahara Kriya

The nature of Higher Consciousness is vibratory. Everything, as we perceive it through our senses, is a manifestation of the oscillations of Nada. Giving into the wisdom of our Higher Mind implies the development of an outer and inner audience so that our sense of listening may become so refined and subtle that it allows us to hear its "dictates" (from Latin "dictare," to dictate, to pronounce solemnly). Deep breathing and deep listening are integral to their mutual efficacy and are beautifully combined in Shabda Pratyahara Kriya.

Shabda Pratyahara Kriya

Here are Swamiji's instructions for this Kriya:

> Sit in any of the recommended postures [comfortable yogic sitting positions] and listen inside of your own head for the subtle sound of blood coursing through the arteries and veins, the sound of blood pressure or the "lub-dub" of the heart's pulsation. Other body sounds may be used as well. Listen intently for two or three minutes, then allow the thinking/hearing to go outside of the body and listen for sounds right around the body. Sometimes a vibrant static sound can be heard in the air immediately around the head. After listening for a few minutes, let the ears come under the control of the mind and listen to your immediate environment to sounds in the room or in the building or in the place where you sit. Now let the hearing go out into the area immediately around the site or building where you sit. Listen to every sound as it occurs. Now reach out with your hearing a hundred meters or so, perhaps up to a city block. Listen to any sounds occurring in that periphery. Stretch out the hearing for a mile, listening to all the sounds circumscribed by the limits of your Pratyahara Kriya. Now, let the thinking/hearing go as far away from you as humanly possible. Concentrating on sending the hearing to far-off distances: listen intently. In this way you have allowed the sense of hearing to do exactly what it has been created to do... to hear. Now having exercised the hearing to its fullest, withdraw the sense of hearing through a reversal of the steps of the Kriya, performing the true purpose of the Pratyahara at each stage until after ten to fifteen minutes, you re-enter the body again. Then listen intently to the subtle sounds within. Raise the mind with the last vestige of this inner concentration on sound into Bhrumadhya or Tisra Til or the Shiva Netra. These centers are included within the concept of Ajna Chakra, the Centre of Inspiration in Tantra, and Kundalini Yoga. ... Be wise enough at this point to recognize the dominant part that the sense of hearing plays in one's Inner Life. In the Inner Life, the senses are reversed. Inner Sight is a lower speed of vibration than Inner Sound. Mastering physical hearing and Shabda, Inner Hearing, is the key to Pratyahara. (Giri, 1976, pp.211–212)

Giving Over: Pranava Pranayama

After cleansing and refining the sense of listening and calming the mind, we are fit to invoke and evoke the powerful Pranava AUM Mantra. The Shabda Pratyahara Kriya prepared us to receive the blessings of such wisdom. The last stage of the Four-Fold Relaxation, Giving Over, completes a cycle of practice that began with the noises of a distracted mind.

Pranava Pranayama

This is one of the gems in the teachings of this Parampara. The practice brings and binds together Asana, Mudra, Pranayama, Pratyahara, and Dharana. The body is held in the Vajra Asana with the Brahma Mudra hand "seal"; the full Mahat Yoga Pranayama is experienced, while the "dance of the tongue" in the oral cavity produces the audible Bija sounds of "AAA," "UUU," and "MMM," starting from the guttural, rising in the palatal, and completing in the cerebral resonators. The mind is focused and calm, one-pointed. The ears and heart open. We offer ourselves to the Divine, which manifests through us through sound, in a sonic embodiment of Nada. When this sequence is complete, we are invited to sit quietly and receive the benefits of a calm mind and an open heart. To come out of such a deep state of relaxation, you may move the pinky of the left hand followed by a gentle movement of the other fingers. You may then decide to lie down in Shava Asana to rest longer or bring the hands into the Namaskara Mudra to intone the Pranava AUM Mantra again to complete the sequence.

This sequence can be practiced every day at the start and end of the day and any time we feel the need to balance our nervous system and quiet the mind. It offers a complete system of centering and rejuvenation, and it helps calm our psychic, emotional, and physical states. It also helps overcome a sense of isolation and fear that may be caused by prolonged distress states. It can be respectfully modified to suit the needs of practitioners, as long as the authenticity of the teachings is not distorted. If properly performed under the guidance of a professionally trained Gitananda Mentor, there are no side effects. Appendix II offers several medical studies on the benefits of these practices.

Blessings for Our Journey Back Home, Sweet OM

Born as a human being, we are endowed with the power of choice.
We can choose our destiny by what we do in the present moment.
Do it now! Do it now! DIN DIN DIN!! said
Swami Gitananda so very often.
If not now, when? If not here, where?
Pujya Ammaji reminds us that Dharma is our responsibility
as a human being to fulfill the purpose of our life, the
purpose of our incarnation of doing the right thing, for the
right person, at the right time, in the right manner.
The *Srimad Bhagavad Gita* reminds us that
the highest Dharma is Swadharma.
The responsibility to our own self is where real Yoga starts.
Nada Yoga enables us to understand the context of the
human incarnation. We understand that we are a spiritual
being enjoying a human experience on planet earth.
Through the Nada Yoga Sadhana, we can attempt to retrace our
way back to the primal source, just like the salmon swims against
the current, moving upstream to go back to its place of birth.
We all have arisen from that causal source of
existence from that Linga/Karana Sharira.
We have manifested through the subtle layers of the Sukshma
Sharira and become the physical entity in this Sthula Sharira. Now
is the opportunity. The present moment, this Kshana provides us

the platform to begin our journey back home, sweet OM. This is a journey that moves from the gross to the causal through the subtle. It is a journey of self, to the Self, through the self. May we all be blessed on this journey. May we all realize our true nature and become one with our innate Divinity. That is our birthright, that is our goal.
Hari Om Tat Sat

To Learn More...

To learn more about Yogamaharishi Dr. Swami Gitananda Giri, the Guru Parampara, and Rishiculture Ashtanga Yoga at Ananda Ashram, ICYER:

www.icyer.com
www.facebook.com/ICYER.Ananda.Ashram

The City Centre of ICYER is called Yoganjali Natyalayam and it was established by Yogamaharishi Dr. Swami Gitananda Giri on March 27, 1993. The flourishing Centre of Classical Rishiculture Yoga, Bharata Natyam, and Carnatic Vocal Music, with currently more than 400 actively enrolled students and more than 20,000 alumni, is located in Central Pondicherry. It caters to the needs of the local populace, with Yoga Education and Yoga Therapy programs, as well as providing special individual and personally tailored lessons for passing tourists and those visiting Pondicherry on a short-term basis:

www.icyer.com/Yoganjali_Natyalayam.htm
www.facebook.com/yognat1993

The Samadhi of the great Guru Dr. Swami Gitananda Giri is located at Sri Kambaliswamy Madam, an ancient Hindu holy site which is the spiritual base of ICYER and its work. Pujas and other cultural and religious festivals are held here:

www.icyer.com/Kambaliswami_Madam.htm
www.facebook.com/SriKambaliswamyMadam

To learn more about Gitananda Nada Yoga, current research, and course offerings:

https://en.soulsound.it/courses/gitananda-nada-yoga
www.facebook.com/groups/gitanandanadayoga
www.instagram.com/gitananda_nada_yoga

To learn more about the medical and scientific research at the Institute of Salutogenesis and Complementary Medicine and the Diplomas in Yoga Therapy and Music Therapy:

www.sbvu.ac.in/iscm

To enroll in online courses with Dr. Ananda Balayogi Bhavanani, including the 52-week *Yoga: Step-by-Step*:

www.icyer.com/Online%20Courses.htm

To purchase books, ebooks, DVDs, and CDs from ICYER:

https://icyer.in

For a list of videos and audio recordings of Gitananda Nada Yoga teachings, practices, research, and cultural events, follow:

Dr. Ananda on social media:
YouTube channel: www.youtube.com/@YogacharyaDrAnandaBhavanani
Facebook: www.facebook.com/ananda.bhavanani

Dr. Sangeeta on social media:
YouTube channel: www.youtube.com/@SangeetaLauraBiagiPhD
Facebook: www.facebook.com/sangeetalaurabiagi

Appendix I

SELECTED MANTRAS AND BHAJANS OF ANANDA ASHRAM/ICYER

Guru Gāyatrī Mantra

ॐ तत् परम्पराय विद्महे |
ज्ञान लिङ्ग ईश्वरय धीमहि
तन्नो गुरुः प्रचोदयात् || ॐ

aum
tat paramparāya vidmahe
jnāna linga ishwaraya (lingeshwaraya) dhimahi
tanno guruh prachodayat
aum

I am aware of the power of the Parampara in my life, the spiritual energy which is available to all of us through the efforts of innumerable Gurus walking the same path, performing the same Sadhana, undergoing the same disciplines. I open myself to that power through the door of the Guru's teaching. I meditate upon that Jnana or wisdom which was achieved by the Guru and now radiates from the Guru's physical symbol (the Samadhi). I open myself to that Guru force. That force of the Universe which dispels the darkness of ignorance and brings the shower of the light of wisdom. May that Guru, that dispeller of darkness, stimulate me and inspire me. May I be worthy of those high teachings. May I be a worthy recipient of this high wisdom.

Gāṇeśa Gāyatrī

ॐ तत् गणेशाय विद्महे
वक्रतुण्डाय धीमहि
तन्नो दंती: प्रचोदयात् || ॐ

aum
tat gaṇeshāya vidmahe
vakra tuṇḍāya dhimahi
tanno daṇtiḥ prachodayāt
aum

I am aware of That Ganesha who is the leader of the Ganas (underworld, netherworld forces). I invoke the One with the twisted trunk (which resembles the shape of the sacred Pranava), this mighty Universal Force Who removes obstacles from all evolutionary undertakings. May I be stimulated and protected by this force.

Subramanyam Gāyatrī

ॐ तत् कुमारय विद्महे
कार्तिकेयय धीमहि
तन्नो स्कन्द प्रचोदयात् || ॐ

aum
tat kumāraya vidmahe
kārtikeyaya dhimahi
tanno skānda prachodayāt
aum

I am aware of the eternally young Kumara, the son of Shiva and Parvati. I meditate upon this universal force which is vibrant, powerful, and able to vanquish all foes with his divine power. That beautiful warrior power I invoke, may it stimulate me.

Sri Durga Gāyatrī

ॐ कात्यायनाय विद्महे |
कन्याकुमारि धीमहि
तन्नो दुर्ग प्रचोदयात् || ॐ

aum
kātyāyanāya vidmahe
kanyākumāri dhimahi
tanno durga prachodayāt
aum

I am aware of the fierce feminine power manifesting as Durga, the powerful Goddess. May She, the pure One, stimulate me to successfully overcome the external and internal negative forces which may come in the way of spiritual evolution!

Sri Lakshmi Gāyatrī

ॐ वरलक्ष्मी च विद्महे
विष्णुपत्नी च धीमहि
तन्नो लक्ष्मी प्रचोदयात || ॐ

aum
varalakshmi cha vidmahe
viṣṇupatni cha dhimahi
tanno lakshmi prachodayāt
aum

I am aware of Lakshmi, She who is the consort of Lord Vishnu, She who is the embodiment of prosperity, well-being, successful endeavors, harmony of the home, well of all those who dwell in our abode. She is the harbinger of good fortune and good luck. I invoke that powerful universal force of prosperity, may it stimulate me.

Sri Sarasvati Gāyatrī

ॐ वीणागणाय विद्महे
विरञ्चपत्नीच धीमहि
तन्नो सरस्वती प्रचोदयात् || ॐ

aum
viṇāgaṇāya vidmahe
viranchapatni cha dhimahi
tanno saraswati prachodayāt
aum

I am aware of She who is the mistress of the musical vina (Vinagana); I invoke Vrinchapatni, who is the consort of Lord Brahma; I invoke She who is the force and power behind divine artistic inspiration and manifestation. I invoke this mighty force, to bless me to manifest the aesthetic impulse of the Universe.

Śivaḥ Gāyatrī

ॐ तन्महेशय विद्महे
वाक् विशुद्धाय धीमहि
तन्न शिव: प्रचोदयात् || ॐ

aum
tan maheśaya vidmahe
vāk viśuddhāya dhimahi
tanna śivaḥḥ prachodayāt
aum

I am aware of that powerful eternal goodness and auspiciousness manifesting as the Divine Lord Shiva. This blue-throated Nilakanta who drank the Hala-Hala poison has the power to purify the voice and the sound with which one expresses oneself. May that eternal goodness inspire me and stimulate me.

Viṣṇu Gāyatrī

ॐ नारायणाय विद्महे
वसुदेवय धीमहि
तन्नो विष्णु प्रचोदयात् || ॐ

aum
nārāyaṇāya vidmahe
vasudevaya dhimahi
tanno viṣṇu prachodayāt
aum

I am aware of that powerful eternal goodness manifesting as Lord Narayana and meditate on the Indwelling Lord of the Universe (Vasu-Deva). May that eternal goodness inspire me and stimulate me.

Lokāḥ Samastāḥ Sukhino Bhavantu (Om Śarve Bhavantu Sukhinah)

ॐ लोकः समस्ताः सुखिनो भवन्तु
सर्वे जनाः सुखिनो भवन्तु
ॐ शान्तिः शान्तिः शान्तिः || ॐ

aum
lokaḥ samastāḥ sukhino bhavantu
sarve janāḥ sukhino bhavantu
om śāntiḥ śāntiḥ śāntiḥ
aum

May all the living beings that exist in all the planes of existence be joyful and be at ease.
May peace manifest at every level of existence.

Selections of Bhajans (ICYER/Ananda Ashram)

Guru Bhajan

ॐ jaya guru om karam jaya jaya
rishi guru om karam om om (x2)
gitananda satguruve satchitananda giri om sharanam (x2)
jaya guru… (x2)
kanakananda satguruve satchitananda giri om sharanam (x2)
jaya guru… (x2)
vivideshananda satguruve satchitananda giri om sharanam (x2)
jaya guru… (x2)
purnananda satguruve satchitananda giri om sharanam (x2)
jaya guru… (x2) ॐ

AUM Victory to you, Guru! The Rishi Guru who
manifests and incarnates the Pranava Om! Victory to you,
Gitananda, the Guru of Truth! Victory to you, Guru!
We bow and salute Guru Kanakananda…
Vivideshananda… Purnananda…
Victory to you, Guru! AUM

Ganesha Bhajan

ॐ ganesha sharanam sharanam ganesha
mahesha sharanam sharanam mahesha
viresha sharanam sharanam viresha
vighnesha sharanam sharanam vighnesha
saisha sharanam sharanam saisha
yogesha sharanam sharanam yogesha ॐ

AUM We bow to You, the Lord of the Ganas
(Gana-Ishwara), we bow to you.
We bow to You, Great Divinity (Maha-Ishwara), we bow to you.
We bow to You, the God of Valor and Vigor
(Vira-Ishwara), we bow to you.
We bow to you, the Remover of Obstacles
(Vighna-Ishwara), we bow to you
We bow to You, Friend of All (Saisha), we bow to you.
We bow to You, Lord of the Yoga (Yoga-Ishwara), we bow to you. AUM

Devi Bhajan

ॐ namostute namostute
jaya sri durga namostute
namostute namostute
jaya sri lakshmi namostute
namostute namostute
jaya sri sarasvati namostute ॐ

AUM We bow to the Resonance of Your Name
(Namostute = namah+astu+te) (x2).
Salutations to you, Sri Durga, salutations!
We bow to the Resonance of Your Name
(Namostute = namah+astu+te) (x2).
Salutations to you, Sri Lakshmi, salutations!
We bow to the Resonance of Your Name
(Namostute = namah+astu+te) (x2).
Salutations to you, Sri Sarasvati, salutations! AUM

Shiva Bhajan

ॐ om namah shivaya (x4)
shiva shiva shiva shiva shiva shivaya (x2)
om namah shivaya (x4)
nama nama nama nama nama shivaya (x2)
om namah shivaya (x4)
adhi adhi adhi adhi adhi shivaya (x2)
om namah shivaya (x4)
para para para para para shivaya (x2)
om namah shivaya (x4)
linga linga linga linga linga shivaya (x2)
om namah shivaya (x4)
nada nada nada nada nada shivaya (x2)
om namah shivaya (x4)
yoga yoga yoga yoga yoga shivaya (x2)
om namah shivaya (x4)
shiva shiva shiva shiva shiva shivaya (x2)
om namah shivaya (x4) ॐ

AUM Salutations to the Divine Self! To the
Supreme Being, Shiva! We bow to you!
We bow to Your Name (nama), to You, the highest (ādhi), to
You, the greatest (para), whose symbol is the Linga (linga), whose
vibration is pure sound (nada), to you, who gifted us with Yoga!
Salutations to the Divine Self! To the Supreme
Being, Shiva! We bow to you! AUM

Vishnu Bhajan

ॐ om namo bhagavate vasudevaya
vasudevaya, vasudevaya, vasudevaya om
vasudevaya, vasudevaya, vasudevaya om ॐ

AUM We bow to Your Effulgence and Benevolence,
Innate Divinity of the Universe,
Innate Divinity of the Universe, We both to You! AUM

Appendix II

ROLE OF YOGA AND MUSIC THERAPIES IN PROMOTING SALUTOGENESIS

Summaries of Research Studies from ISCM, the Institute of Salutogenesis and Complementary Medicine (Previously Known as CYTER and CMTER), Over the Past 15 Years

We offer here the abstracts of a selection of published studies conducted at the Institute of Salutogenesis and Complementary Medicine at Shri Balaji Vidyapeeth, in Pondicherry, India.

Sharma, V. K., Raja, J. M., Velkumary, S., Subramanian, S. K., Bhavanani, A. B., Madanmohan, Sahai, A., & Dinesh, T. (2014). Effect of fast and slow pranayama practice on cognitive functions in healthy volunteers. *Journal of Clinical and Diagnostic Research, 8*(1), 10–13.

Objectives: To compare the cumulative effect of commonly practiced slow and fast pranayama on cognitive functions in healthy volunteers.

Settings and design: 84 participants who were in self-reported good health, who were in the age group of 18–25 years, who were randomized to fast pranayama, slow pranayama and control group with 28 participants in each group.

Material and methods: Fast pranayama included kapalabhati, bhastrika and kukkuriya. Slow pranayama included nadishodhana, pranav and savitri. Respective pranayama training was given for 35 minutes, three times per week, for a duration of 12 weeks under the supervision of a certified yoga trainer. Parameters were recorded before and after 12 weeks of intervention: perceived stress scale (PSS), BMI, waist to hip ratio and cognitive parameters-letter cancellation test, trail making tests A and B, forward and reverse digit spans and auditory and visual reaction times for red light and green light.

Statistical analysis: Inter-group comparison was done by one-way ANOVA and intra-group comparison was done by paired t-test.

Results and conclusion: Executive functions, PSS and reaction time improved significantly in both fast and slow pranayama groups, except reverse digit span, which showed an improvement only in the fast pranayama group. In addition, the percentage reduction in reaction time was significantly more in the fast pranayama group as compared to that in the slow pranayama group. Both types of pranayamas are beneficial for cognitive functions, but fast pranayama has additional effects on executive function of manipulation in auditory working memory, central neural processing and sensory-motor performance.

Bhavanani, A. B., Raj, J. B., Ramanathan, M., & Trakroo, M. (2016). Effect of different pranayamas on respiratory sinus arrhythmia. *Journal of Clinical and Diagnostic Research, 10*(3), CC04–CC06.

Introduction: Respiratory Sinus Arrhythmia (RSA) is the differential change of Heart Rate (HR) in response to inspiration and expiration. This is a non-invasive sensitive index of parasympathetic cardiac control.

Aim: To evaluate changes in RSA by utilizing a simple and cost-effective analysis of electrocardiographic (ECG) tracings obtained during performance of four pranayama techniques.

Materials and methods: Fifty-two trained volunteers performed the following pranayamas with different ratios for inspiration and expiration: sukha (1:1), traditional (1:2), pranava (1:3) and savitri (2:1:2:1), and ECG was recorded while performing the techniques with a rest period of 5 minutes in between. HR was calculated and maximum HR during inspiration (Imax), minimum HR during expiration (Emin), differences between Imax and Emin (Δ), percentage differences between Imax and Emin (Δ%) and expiration: inspiration ratio (E:I) calculated by respective formulae. Statistical analysis was carried out using repeated measures of ANOVA with Tukey-Kramer multiple comparisons test.

Results: There were significant differences between groups in all five aspects, namely: $p = 0.0093$ for mean Imax, $p = 0.0009$ for mean E min, and $p < 0.0001$ for Δ HR (I-E), Δ% HR (I-E) and E:I ratio. Pranava pranayama produced the greatest changes in all five comparisons.

Conclusion: We suggest that further short- and long-term studies be undertaken with pranava pranayama in patients to further qualitatively and quantitatively evaluate inherent mechanisms of this simple technique. Addition of these cost-effective techniques to the medical armory will help patients of rhythm disorders and other cardiovascular conditions.

Bhavanani, A. B., Ramanathan, M., Trakroo, M., & Thirusangu, S. (2016). Effects of a single session of yogic relaxation on cardiovascular parameters in a transgender population. *International Journal of Physiology, 4*(1), 27–31.

Aim and objective: This pilot study was done to determine effects of a single session of yogic relaxation on cardiovascular parameters in a transgender population.

Methods: Heart rate (HR) and blood pressure (BP) measurements were recorded in 106 transgender participants (mean age of 23.86 ± 7.87 y) at the end of a yogic relaxation program at CYTER, MGMCRI. Participants practised a series of techniques consisting of quiet sitting, om chanting, mukhabhastrika, nadishuddhi, brahma mudra, pranava pranayama in sitting posture and savitri pranayama in shavasana. HR and systolic (SP) and diastolic pressure (DP) were recorded before and after the 60-minute session using a non-invasive blood pressure (NIBP) apparatus. Pulse pressure (PP), mean pressure (MP), rate-pressure product (RPP) and double product (DoP) indices were derived from recorded parameters. Student's paired t test was used to compare data that passed normality testing and Wilcoxon matched pairs signed-ranks test for others. P values less than 0.05 were accepted as indicating significant differences for pre-post comparisons.

Results: All recorded cardiovascular parameters witnessed a reduction following the session. This was statistically more significant ($p < 0.0001$) in HR, MP, RPP and DoP and significant ($p = 0.002$) in SP.

Conclusion: There is a healthy reduction in HR, BP and derived cardiovascular indices following a single yogic relaxation session in a transgender population. These changes may be attributed to enhanced harmony of cardiac autonomic function as a result of a mind-body relaxation program. It is suggested that an open and non-hostile environment is conducive for obtaining such a state of psychosomatic relaxation and that such opportunities for transgender participants should be created in all healthcare facilities.

Mathew, D., Sundar, S., Subramaniam, E., & Parmar, P. N. (2017). Music therapy as group singing improves Geriatric Depression Scale score and loneliness in institutionalized geriatric adults with mild depression: A randomized controlled study. *International Journal of Educational and Psychological Researches, 3*(1), 6.

Aims: This study was conducted with an aim to evaluate the effect of group music therapy in the form of group singing, led by a music therapist, on depressive symptoms and loneliness in institutionalized geriatric individuals having mild depression.

Settings and design: The study was conducted as a randomized control trial at St. Mary's Home for the aged, Cuddalore, Tamil Nadu. The study was conducted as a randomized control trial.

Subjects and methods: The experiment group ($n = 40$) received daily music therapy in the form of group singing led by a music therapist for 3 weeks. The control group ($n = 40$) did not receive any specific intervention. Baseline and weekly Geriatric Depression Scale-Short Form (GDS-SF) and UCLA Loneliness Scale scores were recorded in both groups.

Statistical analysis used: Measures of Central Tendency, Mann–Whitney U-test, and Wilcoxon W value.

Results: Statistically significant improvement ($P < 0.05$) was seen in both the scores at the end of 3 weeks in the experiment group as compared to the control group. On intra-group comparison, both scores showed statistically significant improvement ($P < 0.001$) in the experiment group at the end of 3 weeks as compared to baseline but not in the control group. No adverse event was reported.

Conclusions: Group singing significantly improves GDS-SF scores and loneliness in institutionalized geriatric adults having mild depression at the end of 3 weeks. Further research in this area is desirable which could contribute to the well-being of the aged population.

Ajmera, S., Sundar, S., Amirtha, G. B., Bhavanani, A. B., Dayanidy, G., &

Ezhumalai, G. (2018). A comparative study on the effect of music therapy alone and a combination of music and yoga therapies on the psycho-physiological parameters of cardiac patients posted for angiography. *Journal of Basic, Clinical and Applied Health Science, 2,* 163–168.

Background and objectives: Patients undergoing cardiac catheterization and coronary angiography often experience high levels of anxiety and physiological disturbances. Music therapy and music interventions have been found to be effective in bringing down the anxiety and reducing the physiological disturbances for these patients. However, the efficacy of combination of music and yoga therapies for pre-procedural anxiety and physiological disturbances needs to be studied. We aimed in this study to compare the effect of music therapy with the combination of music and yoga therapies to impact the psycho-physiological responses like anxiety, blood pressure, pulse rate and respiratory rate of patients who were posted for coronary angiography.

Material and methods: A total of 45 patients who were posted for coronary angiography were included in the study and randomly divided into three groups. The music therapy group (n = 16) received music listening intervention in the form of listening to pre-recorded, patient-preferred, relaxing raga improvisational music for 15 minutes 1) on the previous day of angiography and 2) 15 minutes before being taken to the catheterization lab on the day of the angiography. The combination of music and the yoga group received both music therapy and yoga therapy in the form of pranava pranayama together for 15 minutes. The control group received only the standard medical treatment. The state of anxiety was measured by a five point single item Likert scale, and the physiological measures such as systolic blood pressure (SBP), diastolic blood pressure (DBP), pulse rate (PR) and respiratory rate (RR) were also recorded for the study.

Results: Both music therapy alone and the combination of music and yoga therapies resulted in significant reduction in anxiety and respiratory rate within the group and the music therapy group recorded additionally significant reduction in SBP, DBP and PR scores during the period of intervention.

Conclusion: Our findings indicate that music therapy alone can bring down the anxiety levels and reduce the physiological disturbances of patients posted for angiography. Also, the combination of music and yoga therapies can bring down the anxiety levels and improve the deep breathing pattern for these patients posted for angiography. More studies are needed to confirm these findings.

Vasundhara, V. R., Bhavanani, A. B., Ramanathan, M., Ghose, S., & Dayanidy, G. (2018). Immediate effect of Sukha Pranayama: A slow and deep breathing technique on maternal and fetal cardiovascular parameters. *Yoga Mimamsa, 50,* 49–52.

Aim: This pilot study was done to evaluate the immediate effect of Sukha Pranayama, a slow and deep breathing technique, on maternal and fetal cardiovascular parameters.

Subjects and methods: Single session pre-post comparison was done for 10 min of Sukha Pranayama in 12 pregnant women in their 3rd trimester. The study participants were guided to breathe in and out in a slow and regular manner for a count of 4 s each. Maternal cardiovascular parameters, namely mean heart rate (MHR), systolic pressure (SP), and diastolic pressure (DP), were measured before and after the session and rate-pressure product (RPP) derived with the formulae. Fetal heart rate (FHR) was derived from the nonstress test tracing.

Results: SP, MHR, FHR, and RPP reduced significantly after a single session of Sukha Pranayama. The mothers reported that they felt more relaxed and also sensed active fetal movement while performing the pranayama.

Discussion: Reduction in maternal cardiovascular parameters may be attributed to reduced sympathetic activity coupled with enhanced vagal parasympathetic tone. Reduction in RPP signifies reduced myocardial oxygen consumption and load on the heart as evidenced by previous studies. These changes in cardiac autonomic status may enhance placental circulation, leading to healthier fetal development.

Conclusion: The present study reiterates the importance of yoga for the psychosomatic health of the maternal-fetal unit as an add-on relaxation technique. We plan to develop this pilot study into a full-fledged evaluation of maternal and fetal wellbeing through yoga.

Raghul, S., Vasanthan, S., Bhavanani, A. B., Jaiganesh, K., & Madanmohan, T. (2018). Effects of overnight sleep deprivation on autonomic function and perceived stress in young health professionals and their reversal through yogic relaxation (Shavasana). *National Journal of Physiology, Pharmacy and Pharmacology*, 8.

Background: Extensive research has been done to demystify the effects of sleep deprivation on cognitive functions, memory, and reasoning ability. However, there is a lacuna in regard to the effects on autonomic function and perceived stress as well as its modulation through yogic relaxation. Health-care professionals often work at night, and the effect of acute overnight sleep deprivation on their performance is crucial.

Aims and objectives: The present study was undertaken to study the effects of overnight sleep deprivation on autonomic function and perceived stress in healthcare professionals and to determine its modulation through yogic relaxation (Shavasana).

Materials and methods: A total of 35 healthcare professionals, aged between 20 and 25 years, were recruited from the emergency services wing (casualty) of MGMC and RI, Puducherry, and taught yogic relaxation. Heart rate (HR), blood pressure (BP), and HR variability (HRV) were recorded and Cohen's perceived stress scale (PSS) administered before the commencement of day duty. Parameters were again recorded after overnight sleep deprivation due to night shift work and then after they practiced yogic relaxation (Shavasana). As data passed normality testing, Student's paired t-test was used to compare the changes after sleep deprivation and then after yogic relaxation.

Results: Overnight sleep deprivation resulted in statistically significant ($P < 0.05$) increases in systolic BP (SBP), low frequency (LF), LF/high frequency (HF), diastolic BP (DBP), PSS, and mean HR. This was coupled with significant decreases in mean RR, SDNN, pNN50, HF, and RMSSD. Following yogic relaxation, these changes were reversed, and significant decreases were witnessed in LF, LF/HF, SBP, mean HR, DBP, and PSS with significant increases in mean RR, pNN50, HF, RMSSD, and SDNN.

Conclusion: The findings of our study reiterate the negative effects of sleep deprivation on cardiac autonomic status. Such deleterious effects may be partially reversed by practicing yogic relaxation (Shavasana). Such conscious relaxation may be able to help correct imbalance of the autonomic nervous system by enhancing parasympathetic tone and reducing sympathetic overactivity.

Ramesh, B., Sundar, S., Jayapreeta, R., Samal, S., & Ghose, S. (2018). Effects of culture-based chants on labour pain during the latent stage of labour in primigravidae mothers: A randomized controlled trial. *Journal of Basic, Clinical and Applied Health Sciences, 2*(1), 16–19.

Background and objectives: Labour is a complex and very painful experience. Poorly relieved pain results in prolonged and stressful labour, maternal impatience in opting for caesarean section and postpartum complications. A positive childbirth experience has a lasting impact on the postpartum health and wellbeing of the new mothers. Music therapy (MT) has been studied to reduce labour pain perception and behaviours and to provide a positive childbirth experience. The study aimed to determine the effect of MT on labour pain and pain behavioural symptoms during the latent stage of labour of primiparous women.

Methods: A total of 120 primiparous women in the latent stage of labour with regular contractions and dilatations less than 4cm were included in the study and randomly divided into two groups. The music group (n = 60) received MT in the form of deep breathing and chanting exercises for one hour between each and every contraction and the control group (n = 60) received only standard treatment. A 10-point visual analogue pain scale (VAS) and Behavioural Pain Rating Scale (BPRS) were measured and recorded by the investigators.

Results: MT intervention resulted in statistically significant reduction in pain and total BPRS scores between the music and the control group with ($p = 0.001$). Also, the BPRS domain scores in facial expression, restlessness, consolation, and vocalization indicated significant reduction due to MT intervention with ($p = 0.001$). The domain of BPRS—muscle tone did not make a significant impact with music.

Conclusion: Chanting and deep breathing experiences as music therapy during the latent stage of labour may reduce pain perception and pain behaviours. Such music therapy interventions may provide positive experiences during childbirth: it could be a safe and dependable method adopted for an effective labour pain management.

Sharma, V. K., Dinesh, T., Rajajeyakumar, M., Grishma, B., & Bhavanani, A. B. (2018). Impact of fast and slow pranayam on cardiovascular autonomic function among healthy young volunteers: Randomized controlled study. *Alternative & Integrative Medicine, 7,* 1000265.

Background: Pranayama refers to the conscious manipulation of the breath in order to modulate the cosmic energy (prana) from the air in the environment. The techniques of pranayam include practices that are performed in a slow or fast type.

Aim: The study aimed to investigate and correlate the impact of three months' practice of fast and slow pranayam on cardiovascular autonomic function among healthy young volunteers.

Materials and methods: A total of 75 volunteer subjects were randomized into a control group (Group 1: n = 25), fast pranayama group (Group 2: n = 25) and a slow pranayama group (Group 3: n = 25). The pranayam practice (Slow Pranayam Group-Savitri, Pranav and Nadisodhana; Fast Pranayam Group-Bhastrika, Kukkuriya and Kapalabhati) was practiced 30 minutes per day, 3 days per week for 3 months either slow or fast pranayam by a certified yoga teacher. The recording of Short-term Heart Rate Variability (HRV) was done at the before and after 3 months of study period.

Result: The LF/HF ratio which is the best indicator of sympatho-vagal balance was reduced significantly in the slow pranayam group showing a shifting of balance towards parasympathetic tone. The RMSSD which is considered to be the best predictor of parasympathetic tone significantly increased in the slow pranayam group. A significant increase (HF) nu and decrease (LF) nu was noted in slow and fast pranayam respectively after yoga intervention.

Conclusion: Results of our study demonstrate that slow and fast pranayam practices are more effective to maintain sympatho-vagal balance by modulating sympathetic and parasympathetic division of the autonomic nervous system.

Abishek, K., Bakshi, S. S., & Bhavanani, A. B. (2019). The efficacy of yogic breathing exercise Bhramari pranayama in relieving symptoms of chronic rhinosinusitis. *International Journal of Yoga, 12*, 120–123.

Introduction: A multitude of modalities are available for the treatment of chronic rhinosinusitis; however, each has its side effects and compliance issues. Bhramari pranayama, which is a breathing exercise in the practice of yoga, offers an inexpensive and free from side effect modality in this regard.

Objective: The objective of this study was to evaluate the efficacy of Bhramari pranayama in relieving the symptoms of chronic sinusitis.

Methodology: A total of 60 patients with chronic sinusitis were randomly divided into two groups: one received conventional treatment of chronic sinusitis and the other group was in addition taught to practice yogic breathing exercise Bhramari pranayama. The patients were advised to practice this breathing exercise twice a day and were followed up at 1, 4, and 12 weeks using the Sino-Nasal Outcome Test (SNOT-22 score).

Results: The mean SNOT-22 score in the group following the Bhramari pranayama breathing exercise using the ANOVA test improved from 39.13 ± 9.10 to 24.79 ± 8.31 (P = 0.0002); this improvement was seen by the end of 4 weeks itself and continued until the 12th week of assessment.

Conclusion: Integrating regular practice of Bhramari pranayama along with the conventional management of chronic rhinosinusitis is more effective than conventional management alone.

Varghese, J. K., Sundar, S., Sarkar, S., & Ezhumalai, G. (2019). Effect of adjuvant music therapy on anxiety, depressive symptoms, and cognitive functions of patients receiving electroconvulsive therapy: A preliminary study. *Journal of Basic Clinical Applied Health Science*, *20*(10), 1–4.

Background and objectives: Electroconvulsive therapy (ECT) is one of the most commonly used treatments for severe psychiatric disorders. Prior and during the ECT treatment, patients may experience varied degrees of anxiety, depressive symptoms, and cognitive impairments. Music therapy (MT) as an adjuvant psychiatric intervention has been successfully employed in many fields of medicine and psychiatry but unexplored in ECT indicative patient groups. This study evaluated the effect of MT on anxiety, depression, and cognitive functions of patients receiving ECT.

Materials and methods: A sample of 29 patients who received ECT as per diagnostic and treatment needs were randomized into cases (n = 14; receiving adjuvant MT) and controls (n = 15; no MT intervention) after subjecting to set criteria. Hospital Anxiety and Depression Scale (HADS) and Montreal Cognitive Assessment (MoCA) were recorded a day before and 15 days after the scheduled four sessions of ECTs were over. Music therapy intervention in the form of Ahir Bhairav raga improvisation, imagery of journey of good health, recovery, and relaxation was administered for cases. Paired t tests and independent t tests were used for intragroup and intergroup comparisons, respectively.

Results: Music therapy intervention resulted in within-the-group significant reduction in anxiety, depression, and improvement in cognitive functioning scores ($p \leq 0.05$). The music therapy group also recorded a significant reduction in total HADS composite scores during the period of intervention.

An intergroup comparison between the MT and the control groups resulted in a significant improvement in anxiety and total HADS scores.

Conclusion: The study results support that MT intervention can be used in clinical settings as an adjunct with ECT, to control anxiety, depression, and cognitive functions in mentally ill patients. More studies with larger sample size are needed to confirm these findings.

Jagadevan, M., Mohanakrishnan, B., Bhavanani, A. B., Shristhudhi, D., Arumugam, P., Subbiah, B., *et al.* (2021). Additive effect of "Brahma Mudra" on pain, proprioception and functional abilities in non-specific mechanical neck pain. *Journal of Bodywork and Movement Therapies, 27,* 717–722.

Objective: Being the second highest musculoskeletal problem irrespective of age, gender and occupation, the etiology of neck pain is predominantly mechanical in nature. This can lead to dysfunction with time and recurrence. Altered joint position sense (JPS) from soft tissues can alter the cervical biomechanics by compromising the cephalo spatial orientation, which depends on the visual, vestibular and proprioceptive cues. This study was done to observe the additive effect of "Brahma mudra" (BM), a yogic tool on non-specific mechanical neck pain and its clinical implication on pain, proprioception and functional abilities.

Methods: It was a quasi-experimental pre-post study design involving 30 individuals from a software firm between the age group of 18 and 45 years. The conventional treatment group received the standard physiotherapy regime and in the BM group BM was incorporated in addition to the standard physiotherapy regime. Independent sample student t-test/Mann Whitney tests were used to compare continuous variables between two groups. Paired sample test/Wilcoxon signed rank tests were used for within groups.

Results: There was a significant reduction in pain and improved functional abilities and proprioception in the BM group when compared to the conventional treatment group with 0.01 level of statistical significance.

Conclusion: It may be concluded that practice of BM had an added effect to the conventional standard physiotherapy regime in reduction of pain and improvement of proprioception and functional abilities among individuals with chronic non-specific mechanical neck pain.

Vasundhara, V. R., Ramanathan, M., Ghose, S., & Bhavanani, A. B. (2022).

Immediate effect of Pranava Pranayama on fetal and maternal cardiovascular parameters. *International Journal of Yoga, 15,* 240–245.

Introduction: Maternal stress responses play an important role in the etiology of fetal and maternal disorders other than biomedical risks. The surge of emergency evidence shows that yoga as an adjuvant therapy can have significant beneficial effects in the prenatal period and in the fetus.

Aim: The aim of this study was to evaluate the immediate effect of Pranava Pranayama on maternal and fetal cardiovascular parameters.

Materials and methods: A three-way cross-over study was done on 3 consecutive days in 60 pregnant women (3rd trimester) with 10 min of breath awareness, listening to OM, and performing Pranava Pranayama. Maternal heart rate (MHR) and systolic and diastolic pressures were measured before and after each session, and cardiovascular indices were derived with formulae. Fetal heart rate (FHR) was obtained from nonstress test tracing. Data were assessed using GraphPad InStat version 3.06. Student's t-test was used for intra-group comparisons while repeated measures ANOVA with Tukey–Kramer multiple comparison tests were done for intergroup comparison.

Results: Significant changes ($P < 0.001$) were found in MHR and FHR immediately after all three interventions. Delta% changes showed the greatest fall in MHR ($P = 0.03$) after Pranava as compared to the other two, while in FHR, both OM group and Pranava were significant ($P < 0.001$).

Conclusion: There were significant changes found in MHR, FHR, and cardiovascular responses rate-pressure product and double product after a single session of intervention. Yogic breathing techniques Pranava may enhance cardiovascular hemodynamics of the maternal–fetal unit. Reduction in maternal and fetal cardiovascular parameters attributed to reduced sympathetic activity coupled with enhanced vagal parasympathetic tone. Such changes in cardiac autonomic status may enhance placental circulation and lead to healthier fetal development.

Ramanathan, M. & Bhavanani, A. B. (2022). Immediate effect of pranava pranayama on oxygen saturation and heart rate in healthy volunteers: A single-blinded, randomized controlled trial. *Medical Journal of Dr. D.Y. Patil Vidyapeeth* [Epub ahead of print]. https://journals.lww.com/mjdy/Abstract/9000/Immediate_Effect_of_Pranava_Pranayama_on_Oxygen.99903.aspx.

Introduction: Yoga is known to promote health and wellness in all.

Pranava Pranayama is a useful sound based yogic breathing technique with reported benefits such as potentiating vagal tone.

Subjects and methods: This single blinded randomized self-controlled cross-over study was done with 58 participants. The immediate effect of Pranava Pranayama on saturation of oxygen in the blood (SpO2) and heart rate (HR) was determined before and after intervention using pulse oximeters. To avoid extraneous influences due to recording on different days, one half of the subjects were randomized to perform quiet sitting on day 1 while the other half did Pranava Pranayama which was then reversed on day 2.

Results: Intra group comparison showed significant changes ($p < 0.001$) in both SpO2 and HR following Pranava Pranayama, whereas in the quiet sitting group, there was an insignificant fall in the SpO2 readings but HR was found to be significant ($p < 0.001$). Intergroup comparison showed significant differences between groups ($p = 0.032$).

Discussion: Cardiovascular changes following Pranava Pranayama may be as a result of audible chanting improving baroreflex sensitivity along with increased endogenous nitric oxide production. This promotes vasodilation resulting in reduction of BP. The decrease in vascular resistance and an increase in capillary perfusion results in increased oxygen saturation with lesser demand on the heart.

Conclusion: This study provides evidence that Pranava Pranayama is an effective technique in enhancing SpO2 and our findings may have therapeutic applications especially in the current pandemic situation.

Appendix III

SELECTED "SATSANGA SHARINGS" BY GITANANDA NADA YOGA MEMBERS

Between December 2021 and June 2022, Dr. Ananda and Dr. Sangeeta led an online Gitananda Nada Yoga Sadhana, a six-month, weekly course whose content inspired the writing of this book. Each week, Dr. Sangeeta prompted the course participants to reflect on some of the topics covered in class and to submit them in a shared document titled "Satsanga Sharing." This Appendix contains a selection of some of these writings first published in two issues of *Yoga Life International Monthly Journal*,[1] as well as unpublished selections from the participants' assignments. The authors have maintained the style and punctuation of the original entries.

1 *Yoga Life International Monthly Journal* is the official publication of: Yoga Jivana Satsangha (International); Vishwa Yoga Samaj (Worldwide Yoga Congress); Sri Kambaliswamy Madam (Samadhi Site); SPARC (The Society for the Preservation of Ancient Rishi Culture); ICYER (International Centre for Yoga Education and Research) at Ananda Ashram, Tamil Nadu. It is published in Ananda Ashram City Centre at Yoganjali Natyalayam, in Pondicherry, India (www.rishiculture.in).

Nada Yoga

First, my heartiest thanks to Dr. Sir AnandaJi and Dr. SangeetaJi for each of your lessons and the practices you shared in the Zoom Womb. The teachings gave a surprising, refreshing, and deeper insight into the ancient science of Nada Yoga, Samkhya, and Tantra. The modern European world is getting senseless and noisier than ever. I was raised without tv, telephone, internet, and without these 50 small noisy electrical machines which, statistically, each householder owns in Germany nowadays. In the 1950s, in Finland, we heard, listened, and acted according to different sounds and voices in the home and in nature. As children, if we wanted to listen to music, we had to sing, and we did! In those times, young children in school learnt by heart the Epic Poem of Finland: Kalevala. The main character is Väinämöinen, the grand epic singer and therapist. He sang: "Mastered by desire impulsive, By a mighty inward urging, I am ready now for singing, Ready to begin the chanting. In my mouth the words are melting, From my lips the tones are gliding, From my tongue they wish to hasten; When my willing teeth are parted, when my ready mouth is opened, Songs of ancient wit and wisdom hasten from me not unwillingly. Come and sing with me the stories, come and chant with me the legends. Since we now are here together, come together from our roamings. Seldom do we come for singing, Seldom to the one, the other..."

At Ananda Ashram, for the first time since my childhood, I heard this "ancient type" of therapeutic singing; Dr. Sir in Kambaliswamy Madam during Pujas or the concerts in the City Center. Unlike Western "emotional" music, this music is structured rhythmically, balancing "waves" deeply inwards. It took several occasions in the Ashram before I re-learnt to hear and listen, to tolerate these vibrations, and to use my own voice more freely.

The Nada Yoga lessons allowed me to experience listening to inner voices, to seek inside of my body the vibrational space for Bijas, Nadis, for Akara-Ukara-Makara and Pranava Aum from bottom of spine upwards to brain, to Trikuthi, and trying to sense the spiraling around the body, to sense movements from left to right side of brain while using Devanagari vowels and consonants loudly and inside my mind, to activate brain structures using lips, teeth, palate and tongue for it.

These teachings nourish our mostly hidden Inner Self, waking up forgotten abilities, entities like SwamiJi Gitananda pointed out: "Wellbeing and Happiness are your birthrights, gain these." Nada Yoga is Tan-Tra! These practices give us the possibility to find the correct distance to our own busy bodies, narcism, give us back the sense of forgotten gift of humor in rush-hour years, and deep relaxation. My best thanks to Divine AmmaJi, who "hit me deeply" (not only) with her incredible sense of humor. P.s. but this is another topic. In gratitude to all Gurus.

Yogacharini Yoga Shakti Latha, Germany

Sāśṭāng praṇāms to Ācārya Dr. Ānanda Bālayōgi Bhavanāni Ji and Saha-Ācārya Dr. Sangītā Laura Biagi Ji. Gītānanda nāda yōga is a pond of ambrosia; or is a sacred river of Gaṅga. Here are people who have come to drink the nectar to their heart's content or to have a holy dip. Most of them have dived into waters, enjoying ecstasy, and are blessed with bliss. A few are standing on the bank, watching the glory of the immersion with awe. But as they cannot remain at the bank standstill, some action sneaks out from them. Without stepping into, leaning and grabbing a handful of water and sprinkling on the head to sanctify and fetching some with both hands together and sipping thrice to make a ritual of Ācamānam. I am one among them.

Dr. Rama Reddy Karri, India

When I breathe [with Sukha Pranayama], I "absorb" Prana, I become aware that the God I'm seeking is right within me. It is my very breath. With every breath, this Divine Potential is manifested within me, and as the Light of the Cosmic Consciousness is flooding through me, I realize I am Sat Chit Ananda. All other senses being dormant, we focus on our auditory perception; becoming aware of all the sounds around us; expanding progressively to the audible vastness. Initially loud, but with practice all external noise sublimate and awareness inverts to the internal sounds. Settling our awareness on the sound of our breath flowing subtly, rhythmically and smoothly much like the Japa Soham. As the mind gets internalized, we progress to the Shanmukhi Mudra with Bhramara/Bhramari Pranayama. A vibration is experienced throughout the head and various colors and patterns emerge in front of the closed eyes. [...] A deep sense of silence and peace is experienced.

Mary Cecil, India

Nada as vibration, Nada in the context of the Pranava AUM, Nada in relation to the Chakras, Nada and Mantras, Bhajans and Carnatic Music, Nada in relation to stress and relaxation, and logically culminating with Nada and Chikitsa. It is nice to focus on one element and revisit the whole through that lens. It forces us to deepen our thoughts and practice within that vista. Revisiting means deepening, making links, studying, contemplating... Any course in the Gitananda tradition would have that impact on any student.

Yogacharya Sri Kant, Canada

A door has been opened to deep learning of the potential impact that Nada, pure vibrational essence of the Universe, can have on self awareness and alleviation of suffering. Understanding Nada, Bindu, Kala as the Causal, Subtle and Gross aspects of reality which govern the processes of manifestation and transformation is foundational. Applying Nada Yoga practices of Kriya and Hatha Yoga such as Shabda Pratyahara, Pranava Pranayama and Pranava OM, we employ somato-psychic mechanisms of refined listening, breath awareness, and vocal sound production, which invoke our intention (through Nama Rupa) to connect with Cosmic Consciousness and evoke potential for positive change. The voice, breath, and mind working together, facilitate understanding and refining of physical senses, then expand beyond to subtle and causal aspects of being by harmonizing and balancing the koshas and enhancing our connection to the chakras, thereby promoting experiences of relaxation and ease, clarity, discernment, and non-attachment, all requirements for well-being of body, mind, and spirit on the conscious journey to freedom and union with Divine vibrational essence. My gratitude for the Gitananda Nada Yoga teachings as shared by Yogacharya Dr. Ananda and Yogacharini Sangeeta is profound.

Michele Wert, USA

Nada Yoga is the rhythm of life. Listen to your heart, your breath, the sound of your voice and the words you choose, the harmonious level of your thoughts. Tune in to the Shabda of the creatures of our natural world who swim, crawl, walk, and fly. Notice when the wind, water, fire, rock, metal, and trees speak. We share a bond of natural biorhythmic connection to Universal Creation, like water flows through the rivers of the earth, and Pranic energy flows through the Nadis. We are connected to each other. Through this connectivity the beauty of our cultural features can be celebrated. In the nurturing environment of this communion, seeds of peacefulness and harmony flourish. The Sadhana of Nada Yoga gives us the ability to perceive the reality of oneness and vibrational connectivity between each and every human being and all aspects of Divine Creation.

Jennifer Kanazawa, British Columbia

Thanks to Nada Yoga we understand the power of vibration and how it is present everywhere in the Cosmos. This vibration can be understood as the pure energy that preceded all Creation: the vibrational essence of the Cosmic Pure Consciousness of Ishvara is the Pranava. It is the combination of Akara Nada, Ukara Nada and Makara Nada coming together in the Omkara. When we want to attune ourselves, the key is the Pranava. I have been practicing Pranava Pranayama for decades and it is always present in my practices. I appreciate the beneficial effects of this practice to manage stress by reducing blood pressure and heart rate. In this course, I found it enlightening to learn the concept that we are able, by using this tool, to reconnect to the Source. When we are aware of how to use Vaikari Nada, we start to realize that we are a vibration of pure Consciousness itself.

Antonio Manzionna, Italy

"The Pranava & the Inner Nada Yoga Journey"

Through Nada Yoga we can attain Self-knowledge. Progress requires sustained practice of authentic yoga teachings and sincere efforts to live those yoga teachings. Through daily practice, sometimes inspired by our tenuous sense of the primordial Pranava vibration, our awareness quietly expands to discover an inner knowing. In the deepest silence, beyond thoughts, we can sense the Pranava vibration as a presence behind the veil. A fleeting intuitive glimpse can start the transformation. In deepest meditations, the silent peace expands and our thoughts slow down. Our mind quiets. Our awareness, as if seated somewhere far away from life's dramas, feels the Pranava. Eventually our silent seat develops deeper roots in an enduring silence that expands beyond all measures.

The teaching is of Transformation. The drop merges into the ocean. We surrender our finite limited identity as the transformation proceeds through a threshold between the subtlest layers of manifest creation and the un-manifest non-dual source of all. We chant, focus and attune to the Pranava and grasp at the Pranava sound as a sacred thread to guide our inner journey. The inner Nada Yoga practices are essential enablers on this journey. On the other side of vast silence, total stillness, the Pranava is waiting for us there. The Pranava is the gateway to the vastness, the stillness beyond dualities, beyond dimensionality. Some call it the void. For me, it seems more of a fullness. A fullness of being-ness. Said to be ineffable. Our words are insufficient.

Yogacharya Bharata Bill Francis Barry, USA

Reflections on the Pranava Aum[2]

"The Direct Journey Home: Pranava AUM"

From the manifest to the unmanifest
From the mundane to the spiritual
From the profane to the profound
From the worldly to the sacred
From the seen to the unseen
From the heard to the unheard
From the imagined to what lies beyond imagination
From the conceived to what cannot be conceived
From what is known to the landscape of the unknown
From what is possible to the realm that holds all possibilities
From Sthula to Karana
From Jagrat to Turiya Atita
From Vishwa to Pragnya
From being enmeshed in the dance of Gunas
to the Kaivalya of Guna Atita
From Nara to Narayana
To that Akara Ukara Makara Omkara Roopinin Ambe
I prostrate before and offer my humble salutations.

Shailaja Menon, Malaysia

I sit.
With "O Heavenly King," devotion I bring. Amin!
With Mukha Bhastrika, the temple is cleaned,
With Vibhaga and Sparsha, the light turns on within.

2 First published in *Yoga Life International Monthly Journal*, 53(3), 20–26.

Akara and Chin—the lower comes alive!
Ukara and Chinmaya—the mid revives!
Makara and Adhi—high five!
Now the temple is open, clear and clean.
The gesture of God I bring in,
I bow and surrender within,
I invoke the Divine to come in:
AUM, AUM, AUM, AUM, AUM, AUM!
Amin and AUM, brought the Divine in?
The after-effect is silence within.
Now, what is "within" and who is sitting?

Ovidiu Ponoran, Romania

Feeling my body,
sensitive sensual touch.
Front-side-back, back-side-front.
Expanding, pulsating, vibrating, softening, slowing down, grounding.
Breathe deeply, inhale-exhale, inhale-exhale.
Counting, structured.
Give up control, finding my own rhythm.
Listen to my voice, unsure, shaking, uneven and flipping.
Adjust, refine, grow in trust.
Expressing who I am; loving without judgment.
Feel the Divine Prana,
life giving, live sustaining,
buzzing, tingling, healing, nurturing. Warm and golden.
Flows through me, my breath, my voice.
Each incantation unique in expression,
perfectly imperfect, just like we are.
Falling in love with AUM.
Rising in AUM
Listen to the Silence.
That Is. That Was. That Will be. Always. Everywhere.
Pranava AUM.
Vehicle and Destination.

Hwamin Fettes, Australia

Who holds my life in warm, solid earthed-
hands, anchors it in oaken-roots.
Mother—Ahhh—Guttural, resonant as she gave birth to all of creation.
Son, the OOH—the music I make, the love and expansiveness
in my heart as faces soften with words and melody. My arms
reach and embrace the Tree. Resting my cheek on the roughened
bark, my heart opens in receipt of love. Christ in all creation.
Divine Spirit—mmmm. Delicious and pure. Breath and fire. Reaching
skyward, flowing water. I can almost feel the life force in you as it
moves upwards in Winter branches whispering Three-In-One.

Bridget Hamill, Northern Ireland

I love chanting the Pranava, and this has been wonderfully
enhanced by the incorporation of the Hasta Mudras.
I love the way it shifts my physical boundaries and
I feel as if I have had "an inner shower."
It opens me up to a shimmering stillness and spaciousness. I
am drawn into an ever-widening hoop of silence, with the inner
and outer phenomena 'somewhere out there' on the rim.
In the center, or hub, I simply abide in the sacred
presence; there is just the vibration of the heart,
chanting Japa on my behalf: "OM, OM, OM…"
My teacher taught me, as I in turn teach others, to
visualize the Pranava as "growing your lotus."
The mud at the bottom of the lake is the world of Prakriti,
with all our experiences, conditioning and Karma.
The "A" sound represents our roots in this world of matter, which
nourish and sustain us, but out of which we must evolve.
The "U" sound is the stem, our spiritual sadhana, our
journey upwards through the dark lake waters.
The "M" sound is when our little bud / buddhi emerges
and awakens to the light of higher awareness.
The fourth stage is abidance in the underlying silence, with
the petals of our lotus fully opened to the Spiritual Sun.
The mud, the roots, the stem, the flower and the sun are all one.
Om Tat Sat.

Yogacharya Michael McCann, Northern Ireland

Pranava Aum
Where would I be without you
You ground me
You center me
You calm me
You ignite me
You focus me
You are the eternal sound
You are the breath
You are the link
You are the cosmos
Without you I would lose myself Back to the world of man.

Amanda Paulson, Canada

Inhale
Low Mid Upper
Akara, Ukara, Makara
Exhale, Low Mid Upper. Silence
Resonance. At first it is mechanical
And then something takes over. Warmth
Felt through the body. The sound of other voices
All around me, students following their own metronome
Breath, sound, vibration. Connecting to the universe. Cosmic Life force
A journey to uncover the True Self with universal vibration and energy
Otherworldly sounds making their way into the consciousness
A feeling of non-duality. Homecoming. Calm. Peace
A spiral of energy outward and upward and
Then, surrender inward and elevated
Time is seemingly standing still
This is the practice of Pranava
That which preceded all
Manifestation
AUM

Shell Andrea, Canada

Ammaji told me: "If you can't chant
AUM as long as the others,

Just sense the areas being activated
By the vibrations." So I did,
Becoming very involved and acquainted with
the geography of my lungs. Then,
There was mathematics to consider: how long to allot to each section
Of each lobe of each lung.
Quickly I mastered pulmonary
mathematical geography.
To help others I proposed assorted Images to keep them on the
Right trail in the right direction.
But the day Dr. Sir and
Sangeeta talked of the Nâda rolling
Up, along, and up changed my
Whole perception! Just follow the Nâda From Manipûra to the heavens!

Yogacharini Yogashakti Yogachemmal Jnānasundarī, France

Pranava Om am I
Experiencing Infinity
Carrying all your Mind, Spirit and Body
Am the bridge
The channel to the Divine
Pranava Pranayama am I
Symphony of Om-Karas
Akara Ukara Makara
Vibhaga Pranayama am I
Every lung lobe I envelop
Vyaghra Pranayama am I
Like a fearless tiger
Keeping your spine strong
Let's dance in harmony
Kaya Kriya am I
Expelling your past physical body traumas
Mahat Yoga Pranayama am I
Balancing Prana and Apana
Comprising all three
Adam Pranayama Akara
Always Chin Mudra

Madhya Pranayama Ukara
Always Chinmaya Mudra
Adhyam Pranayama Makara
Always Adhi Mudra
So come everybody
Let's learn and do
Am always with you.

Smita Benny, India

I am peering into a vast sacred cavern pulsing with millions of sparks of pure, white light.
Here is the abode of the Divine,
the Cosmic Life Force.
Seated in Vajrasana, with each mindful breath
the pure white light of divinity arises from the depths of my being
and spirals upwards tracing the sacred symbol of Om.
The Divine Prana is pulsing through me, vibrating
with the sound of the PranavaAUM.
With each inspiration my attention is drawn inwards
(Puraka) as I hold the sacred breath (Kumbhaka), exhaling
(Rechaka) as I surrender the ego and contemplate the silence
(Shunyaka). My body a temple of the Holy Spirit.

Margaret O'Neill, Northern Ireland

The vibration of AUM, a central element in Nada Yoga—the Yoga of sound and vibration—is impacting your body and your mind. The sound of Aum, following and prolonging your outbreath. First Adham, then Madhyam, and finally Adhyam. Breathe in, filling every section of your lungs. Breathe out, let the AUM prolong your breath, create vibration, for your intense being in the Universe.

Ingunn Hagen, Norway

Satsanga Sharings on Stress and Yoga[3]

Pwy sau is the Welsh word for stress, the root of which comes from the word "pwys," meaning weight. Stress to me is when you are burdened with an overwhelming "weight" that does not shift and is nigh impossible to off-load. It is like a length of wire tensioned so tightly at both ends that it is close to breaking point. That tension is almost palpable. Stress is something that has hit each and every one of us, most likely on a daily basis since the start of the pandemic. [...] A lot of people did change the way they looked at this precious planet that we call home. The lungs of Mother Earth were starting to breathe properly, into all lobes, front, back and sides. [...] The crisis, as many see it, is over—which of course it isn't. I think most of the stress in my life right now is born of frustration knowing that things are reverting back to the ME, ME, ME... the reflection that Covid mirrored for us was the WE, WE, WE and how good that felt. A lot of that community spirit is now disappearing along with face masks and PCR testing, like it had all been a bad dream. To me, the current situation presents with more stress than any lockdown.

Yoga is my lifeboat that keeps me afloat through the good and the downright dreadful. On a good day I get to see the beautiful, blue ocean as I bob across its surface. My lungs are filled with prana as I take in the clean, ozone filled air. I am lifted. But when I can see the storm clouds gathering on the horizon I know that my Yoga, my life boat, will help me hold fast, in body, mind and spirit. Just me, my boat, my Yoga and no tigers.

Jan Hallé, UK

Stress is a compression cum oppression. Stress is reactionary and volatile in nature. Stress reduces our ability to choose and to be more responsible. Stress decreases our efficient growth of easiness and leads us to dis-ease. It is like a traffic jam where one is bound to pollute in all ways. But the power of choice to turn off the engine for some time gives us a clarity of finding peace within despite the external or internal pressure of thoughts, irritability, dislike, hatred, tiredness and modern-day frustrations.

Some of my current stressors are around womanhood experiences. Since I have gained consciousness being a girl, a teen, a woman, a daughter, a wife, a mother, I have seen that we have to always do more to be able to survive

3 First published in *Yoga Life International Monthly Journal*, *53*(7), 18–21.

in this so-called gender equal society. It's always very disappointing to hear the stories of amazing women who have done so much to this world and society, but their strong images and credits just diminish under the title of a secondary class. I have seen how the minorities face challenges just to get an average paid job to be a counterpart in the dominant world society of survival of the fittest. When we teach our new young generation the equality of rights and freedom to make choices, it often becomes more like a statement than a deed or action in society. Life itself is very challenging in these times. So, it is more important to be emotionally constructive and well nourished at physical and mental levels. In this way, we need hand in hand to be safe and be in a rest and digest state to perform our responsibilities for a better tomorrow.

Yoga helps me to cope with these man-made differences through various powerful statements taught by Yoga Acharya Dr. Anandaji. "Do your best and leave the rest! Everyone has their own Swadharma and the approach of Swadhyaya." So, when I listen to such amazing statements, I am constantly thankful to this lineage for accepting us as we are! And, giving us courage to be the best version of one's own self.

Gurleen Sarai, Canada

Gratitude

"Thank you" is a word of immense depth, beauty and harmony.

"Thank you," even before it is an audible sound, it is a vibration within us, and the reason why directing as many thoughts and words of kindness to others gives care and kindness to our cells, our organs, our heart. I learned the concept of Nāma-Rūpa—word vibration—during the Gitananda Nada Yoga Immersion course. Nāma refers to the vibration of the word we pronounce. Rūpa is the form of the vibration we pronounce. This is why I find the energy of the word THANK YOU wonderful. The energy of this simple but powerful word, in vibrating it, loosens all tensions and harmonizes with the Whole.

And it is with this vibration that I wish to express my gratitude to Dr. Ananda and Dr. Sangeeta, THANK YOU.

Caterina Caizzone, Italy

Bibliography and Other Resources

Abishek, K., Bakshi, S. S., & Bhavanani, A. B. (2019). The efficacy of yogic breathing exercise Bhramari pranayama in relieving symptoms of chronic rhinosinusitis. *International Journal of Yoga, 12*, 120–123.

Ajmera, S., Sundar, S., Amirtha Ganesh, B., Bhavanani, A. B., Dayanidy, G., & Ezhumalai, G. (2018). A comparative study on the effect of music therapy alone and a combination of music and yoga therapies on the psycho-physiological parameters of cardiac patients posted for angiography. *Journal of Basic, Clinical and Applied Health Science, 2*, 163–168.

Antonovsky, A. (1979). *Health, stress and coping.* Jossey-Bass.

Antonovsky, A. (1987). *Unraveling the mystery of health: How people manage stress and stay well.* Jossey-Bass.

Appleton, J. (2018). The gut-brain axis: Influence of microbiota on mood and mental health. *Integrative Medicine: A Clinician's Journal, 17*(4), 28–32.

Beck, G. L. (2009). *Sonic theology: Hinduism and sacred sound.* University of Carolina Press.

Benson, H. (1975). *The relaxation response.* William Morrow.

Berendt, J. E. (1993). *The world is sound: Nada Brahma.* Destiny Books.

Bernardi, L., Sleight, P., Bandinelli, G., Cencetti, S., Fattorini, L., Wdowczyc-Szulc, J., & Lagi, A. (2001). Effect of rosary prayer and yoga mantras on autonomic cardiovascular rhythms: Comparative study. *British Medical Journal, 323*(7327), 1446–1449.

Bhavanani, A. B. (2002). *A primer of yoga theory for yoga sports, yoga teachers and yoga students.* Dhivyananda Creations.

Bhavanani, A. B. (2003). *A yogic approach to stress: Based on Gitananda Yoga teachings in the tradition of Rishiculture Ashtanga Yoga.* Satya Press.

Bhavanani, A. B. (2005). *Yoga 1 to 10: Understanding yogic concepts through a numerical codification.* Satya Press.

Bhavanani, A. B. (2007). *Yoga therapy notes.* Dhivyananda Creations.

Bhavanani, A. B. (2008a). *Chakras: The psychic centers of yoga and tantra.* Dhivyananda Creations.

Bhavanani, A. B. (2008b). *Yoga for health and healing.* Dhivyananda Creations.

Bhavanani, A. B. (2011a). *Understanding the yoga darshan: An exploration of the yoga sutra by Maharishi Patanjali.* Dhivyananda Creations.

Bhavanani, A. B. (2011b). *Chanting the yoga sutras* [CD]. Geetanjali Super Audio (Madras).

Bhavanani, A. B. (2013a). *Yoga chikitsa: Applications of yoga as a therapy.* Dhivyananda Creations.

Bhavanani, A. B. (2013b). *Psychosomatic mechanisms of yoga* [CME-cum-Workshop presentation]. Yoga & Lifestyle Disorders, Department of Physiology and Centre for Yoga Therapy, Education and Research (CYTER), Mahatma Gandhi Medical College & Research Institute (MGMC&RI), 29–43.

Bhavanani, A. B. (2017). Role of yoga in prevention and management of lifestyle disorders. *Yoga Mīmāṃsā, 49*, 42–47.

Bhavanani, A. B. (2022). *Dr Anandaji on the "12 Chakra Concept" of Rishiculture Gitananda Yoga in Scintillating Saturdays #95* [Video]. https://youtu.be/jtzAMl_2K3s.

Bhavanani, A. B. & Biagi, S. L. (2013). *Saraswati's pearls: Dialogues on the yoga of sound.* Dhivyananda Creations.

Bhavanani, A. B. & Biagi, S. L. (2021). *Perle di SARASVATĪ: Dialoghi sullo yoga del suono.* Lakṣmi Edizioni.

Bhavanani, A. B., Madanmohan, & Sanjay, Z. (2012a). Immediate effect of chandra nadi pranayama (left unilateral forced nostril breathing) on cardiovascular parameters in hypertensive patients. *International Journal of Yoga, 5*(2), 108–111.

Bhavanani, A. B., Madanmohan, & Sanjay, Z. (2012b). Suryanadi pranayama (right unilateral nostril breathing) may be safe for hypertensives. *Journal of Yoga & Physical Therapy, 2*, 118.

Bhavanani, A. B., Madanmohan, Sanjay, Z., & Basavaraddi, I. V. (2012). Immediate cardiovascular effects of pranava pranayama in hypertensive patients. *Indian Journal of Physiology and Pharmacology, 56*(3), 273–278.

Bhavanani, A. B., Madanmohan, Zeena, S., & Vithiyalakshmi, L. (2012). Immediate cardiovascular effects of pranava relaxation in patients with hypertension and diabetes. *Biomedical Human Kinetics, 4*, 66–69.

Bhavanani, A. B., Malini, Y., & Padma, Y. (2021). *Yoga and Cultural Misappropriation.* ICYER. https://icyer.in/product/yoga-and-cultural-misappropriation.

Bhavanani, A. B., Raj, J. B., Ramanathan, M., & Trakroo, M. (2016). Effect of different pranayamas on respiratory sinus arrhythmia. *Journal of Clinical and Diagnostic Research, 10*(3), CC04–CC06.

Bhavanani, A. B. & Ramanathan, M. (2012). Immediate cardiovascular effects of savitri pranayama in sitting and supine positions in female volunteers. *Yoga Mimamsa, 44*, 101–112.

Bhavanani, A. B., Ramanathan, M., Balaji, R., & Pushpa, D. (2013). Immediate effect of suryanamaskar on reaction time and heart rate in female volunteers. *Indian Journal of Physiology Pharmacology*, *57*(2), 199–204.

Bhavanani, A. B., Ramanathan, M., Balaji, R., & Pushpa, D. (2014a). Differential effects of uninostril and alternate nostril pranayamas on cardiovascular parameters and reaction time. *International Journal of Yoga*, *7*, 60–65.

Bhavanani, A. B., Ramanathan, M., Balaji, R., & Pushpa, D. (2014b). Comparative immediate effect of different yoga asanas on heart rate and blood pressure in healthy young volunteers. *International Journal of Yoga*, *7*, 89–95.

Bhavanani, A. B., Ramanathan, M., & Madanmohan. (2013). Immediate cardiovascular effects of a single yoga session in different conditions. *Alternative & Integrative Medicine*, *2*, 144.

Bhavanani, A. B., Ramanathan, M., & Madanmohan. (2014). Immediate effect of alternate nostril breathing on cardiovascular parameters and reaction time [Special Issue]. *Online International Interdisciplinary Research Journal*, *4*, 297–302.

Bhavanani, A. B., Ramanathan, M., Trakroo, M., & Thirusangu, S. (2016). Effects of a single session of yogic relaxation on cardiovascular parameters in a transgender population. *International Journal of Physiology*, *4*(1), 27–31.

Bhavanani, A. B., Sanjay, Z., & Madanmohan. (2011). Immediate effect of sukha pranayama on cardiovascular variables in patients of hypertension. *International Journal of Yoga Therapy*, *21*, 73–76.

Bhavanani, M. D. (1984). *Yoga: One woman's view*. Satya Press.

Biagi, S. L. (2018). *Reimagine failure: Breathe, belong, believe* [TEDx Talks]. TEDx DePaul University. www.ted.com/talks/laura_biagi_reimagine_failure_breathe_belong_believe.

Biagi, S. L. (2021). *La voce arcana: Viaggio alla scoperta di Sé attraverso gli Arcani Maggiori dei Tarocchi*. RP Libri.

Biagi, S. L. & Conti, M. R. (2022, Giugno). Arte del respiro. *Yoga Journal Italia*, 41–47.

Dhar, N., Chaturvedi, S. K., & Nandan, D. (2013). Spiritual health, the fourth dimension: A public health perspective. *WHO South-East Asia Journal of Public Health*, *2*, 3–5.

Digambarji, S. & Gharote, M. L. (Eds.). (1997). *Gheraṇḍa Saṃhitā*. Kaivalyadhama S.M.Y.M. Samiti.

Feuerstein, G. (1998). *Tantra: The path of ecstasy*. Shambhala Press.

Frawley, D. (2010). *Mantra Yoga and Primal Sound: Secrets of Seed (Bija) Mantras*. Lotus Press.

Giri, G. S. (1976). *Yoga: Step-by-step*. Satya Press.

Giri, G. S. (1984). *Swamiji 12 Chakras, Part 2* [Video]. https://youtu.be/uN0fGwzn6NI.

Giri, G. S. (1995). *Yantra: The mystic science of number, name and form*. Satya Press.

Giri, G. S. (2008). *Pranayama: The fourth limb of Ashtanga Yoga*. Satya Press.

Giri, G. S. (2022). Rudraksha—the Tears of Shiva. *Yoga Life International Monthly Journal*, *53*, 6, 10–23.

Giri, G. S. (n.d.) Tuning into the universe one-pointedness with the primordial sound-Aum. www.icyer.com/documents/Swamiji_pranava_article.pdf.

Giri, G. S. & Bhavanani, A. B. (2008). *Yoga for breathing disorders.* Dhivyananda Creations.

Jagadevan, M., Mohanakrishnan, B., Bhavanani, A. B., Shristhudhi, D., Arumugam, P., Subbiah, B., *et al.* (2021). Additive effect of brahma mudra on pain, proprioception and functional abilities in non-specific mechanical neck pain. *Journal of Bodywork and Movement Therapies, 27*, 717–722.

Jenny, H. (1967). *Cymatics: A study of wave phenomena and vibration.* Basilius.

Johari, H. (2000). *Chakras: Energy centers of transformation.* Destiny Books.

Khan, H. I. K. (1996). *The mysticism of sound and music.* Shambhala Dragon Editions.

Krishnakumar, D., Hamblin, M. R., & Lakshmanan. (2015). Meditation and yoga can modulate brain mechanisms that affect behavior and anxiety: A modern scientific perspective. *Ancient Science, 2*(1), 13–19.

Lokeswarananda, S. (1993). *Kāṭha Upaniṣad: Translated and with notes based on Śaṅkara's commentary.* The Ramakrishna Mission Institute of Culture.

Lokeswarananda, S. (1995). *Māṇḍūkya Upaniṣad: With Gauḍapāda's kārikā.* The Ramakrishna Mission Institute of Culture.

Madanmohan, Bhavanani, A. B., Dayanidy, G., Sanjay, Z., & Basavaraddi, I. V. (2012). Effect of yoga therapy on reaction time, biochemical parameters and wellness score of peri and postmenopausal diabetic patients. *International Journal of Yoga, 5*(1), 10–15.

Madanmohan, Bhavanani, A. B., Sanjay, Z., Vithiyalakshmi, L., & Dayanidy, G. (2013). Effects of a comprehensive eight week yoga therapy programme on cardiovascular health in patients of essential hypertension. *Indian Journal of Traditional Knowledge, 12*, 535–541.

Madanmohan, Thombre, D. P., Das, A. K., Subramanian, N., & Chandrasekar, S. (1984). Reaction time in clinical diabetes mellitus. *Indian Journal of Physiology and Pharmacology, 28*(4), 311–314.

Mathew, D., Sundar, S., Subramaniam, E., & Parmar, P. N. (2017). Music therapy as group singing improves Geriatric Depression Scale score and loneliness in institutionalized geriatric adults with mild depression: A randomized controlled study. *International Journal of Educational and Psychological Researches, 3*(1), 6.

Muktibodhananda, Swami. (1998). *Hatha yoga pradipika, under the guidance of Swami Satyananda Saraswati.* Bihar School of Yoga.

Nagarajan, K. (2021). *An introduction to Indian music therapy.* Author Vine.

NASA Space Place (2023). What Is the Big Bang? https://spaceplace.nasa.gov/big-bang/en.

1 Girl Revolution (Director). (2020). *The Girl Inside* [Video]. Behold. https://youtu.be/v583zIwMKeE.

Padoux, A. (1990). *Vāc: The concept of the word in selected Hindu tantras* (J. Gontier, Trans.). State University of New York Press.

Padoux, A. (2011). *Tantric mantras: Studies on mantrasastra.* Routledge.

Padoux, A. (2017). *The Hindu tantric world: An overview.* University of Chicago Press.

Parthasarathi, S. K. (2020). Ancient science of mantras—Wisdom of the sages. *International Journal of Yoga, 13*(1), 84–86.

Prabhupāda, A. C. B. S. (1986). *Bhagavad-gītā as it is.* The Bhaktivedanta Book Trust.

Pramanik, T., Pudasaini, B., & Prajapati, R. (2010). Immediate effect of slow pace breathing exercise bhramari pranayama on blood pressure and heart rate. *Nepal Medical College Journal, 12,* 154–157.

Raghul, S., Vasanthan, S., Bhavanani, A. B., Jaiganesh, K., & Madanmohan, T. (2018). Effects of overnight sleep deprivation on autonomic function and perceived stress in young health professionals and their reversal through yogic relaxation (Shavasana). *National Journal of Physiology, Pharmacy and Pharmacology, 8.*

Ramanathan, M. & Bhavanani, A. B. (2014). Immediate effect of chandra and suryanadi pranayamas on cardiovascular parameters and reaction time in a geriatric population. *International Journal of Physiology, 2*(1), 59–63.

Ramanathan, M. & Bhavanani, A. B. (2022). Immediate effect of pranava pranayama on oxygen saturation and heart rate in healthy volunteers: A single-blinded, randomized controlled trial. *Medical Journal of Dr. D.Y. Patil Vidyapeeth.* [Epub ahead of print]. https://journals.lww.com/mjdy/Abstract/9000/Immediate_Effect_of_Pranava_Pranayama_on_Oxygen.99903.aspx.

Ramanathan, M., Bhavanani, A. B., & Trakroo, M. (2017). Effect of a 12-week yoga therapy program on mental health status in elderly women inmates of a hospice. *International Journal of Yoga, 10*(1), 24–28.

Ramesh, B., Sundar, S., Jayapreeta, R., Samal, S., & Ghose, S. (2018). Effects of culture-based chants on labour pain during the latent stage of labour in primigravidae mothers: A randomized controlled trial. *Journal of Basic, Clinical and Applied Health Sciences, 2*(1), 16–19.

Saraswati, S. C. (2009). *The Vedas.* Bharatiya Vidya Bhavan.

Sharma, V. K., Dinesh, T., Rajajeyakumar, M., Grishma, B., & Bhavanani, A. B. (2018). Impact of fast and slow pranayam on cardiovascular autonomic function among healthy young volunteers: Randomized controlled study. *Alternative & Integrative Medicine, 7*(2), 1–6.

Sharma, V. K., Raja Jeyakumar, M., Velkumary, S., Subramanian, S. K., Bhavanani, A. B., Madanmohan, & Dinesh, T. (2014). Effect of fast and slow pranayama practice on cognitive functions in healthy volunteers. *Journal of Clinical and Diagnostic Research, 8*(1), 10–13.

Sobana, R., Jaiganesh, K., & Barathi, P. (2013a). Role of Rag Ahir Bhairav as complementary and alternative medicine (CAM) on blood pressure in prehypertensive adults. *Journal of Medical Science and Technology, 2*(2), 66–70.

Sobana, R., Jaiganesh, K., & Bharathi, P. (2013b). A study on the relationship of music therapy and personality traits of neuroticism and agreeableness. *National Journal of Research in Community Medicine, 2*(1), 1–78.

Thiruvalluvan, A., Sekizhar, V., Ramanathan, M., Bhavanani, A. B., Chakravathy, D., & Reddy, J. R. C. (2021). Effect of pranayama techniques with marmanasthanam kriya as yogic relaxation on biopsychosocial parameters prior to endodontic therapy: A cross sectional study. *International Journal of Yoga, 14*, 146–151.

Varghese, J. K., Sundar, S., Sarkar, S., & Ezhumalai, G. (2019). Effect of adjuvant music therapy on anxiety, depressive symptoms, and cognitive functions of patients receiving electroconvulsive therapy: A preliminary study. *Journal of Basic Clinical Applied Health Science, 20*(10), 1–4.

Vasundhara, V. R., Bhavanani, A. B., Ramanathan, M., Ghose, S., & Dayanidy, G. (2018). Immediate effect of sukha pranayama: A slow and deep breathing technique on maternal and fetal cardiovascular parameters. *Yoga Mimamsa, 50*, 49–52.

Vasundhara, V. R., Ramanathan, M., Ghose, S., & Bhavanani, A. B. (2022). Immediate effect of pranava pranayama on fetal and maternal cardiovascular parameters. *International Journal of Yoga, 15*, 240–245.

Venkatesananda, S. (2007). *The supreme yoga: Yoga vashista.* Motilal Banarsidass Publishers.

Vialatte, F. B., Hovagim, B., Rajkishore, P., & Cichocki, A. (2009). EEG paroxysmal gamma waves during bhramari pranayama: A yoga breathing technique. *Consciousness and Cognition, 18*, 977–988.

Weitzberg, E. & Lundberg, J. (2002). Humming greatly increases nasal nitric oxide. *American Journal of Respiratory and Critical Care Medicine, 166*(2), 144–145.

WHO (2023). Constitution. www.who.int/about/governance/constitution.

Woodroffe, J. (2009). *The serpent power: Being the ṣaṭ-cakra-nirūpaṇa and pādukā-pañcaka.* Ganesh and Company.

Yoga Life International Monthly Journal: The official publication of Yoga Jivana Satsangha (International). Bhavanani, M. D. (Ed.). Ananda Ashram City Centre, Yoganjali Natyalayam.

Yogananda, Paramahansa. (1995). "God talks with Arjuna." In *The Bhagavad Gita: Volume I.* Self Realization Fellowship.

Index